DEAR OPRAH

The Health Book for Everyone!

by Dr. Dale Ellwein

My interpretations and conclusions contained in this book come from my 20 plus years of experience as a health professional helping patients, with similar health fluctuations to Oprah Winfrey's. I have found that, with the methods written in this book, my patients achieve the health and life of their dreams.

This book's contents and the cover are not endorsed by Oprah Winfrey (as of yet).

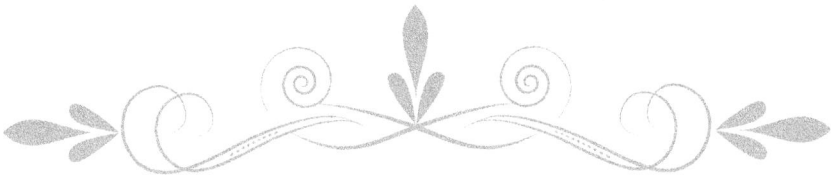

I dedicate this book to all those who have had or have health challenges and to those who have been looking for true health answers. My wish is for you to find hope within these pages and uncover the drive to make the lasting changes for the best life possible.

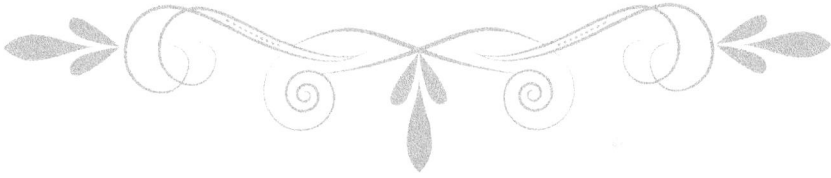

Table of Contents

Health means having the energy and stamina to do what you want to do when you want to do it.

Dr. Dale Ellwein

Acknowledgments

I wish to acknowledge the following people for their support and assistance in the creation of this book:

- My wife, Barbara, and my children, Evan and Jace—the loves of my life—and my motivation to be and do my best.

- Dr. James L. Chestnut for inspiring me with the genius of his teachings of the true wellness lifestyle which I refer to often throughout this book. You have been an amazing influence on my life and practice.

- Dr. Pat Gentempo and Creating Wellness Alliance for the scientific representation of wellness.

- Dr. Russ Rosen, Drs. Barry Anderson and Daniel Bai from Everest Coaching Systems, Drs. Larry, Bob, and Dennis from the Masters Circle, Dr. Steve Hoffman, Dr. Mark Kimes, and Dr. Scott Sawyer, all of my chiropractic coaches throughout my career, for keeping me on track in helping humanity.

- Susan Stroh, my writing partner and coach, who kept me focused and showing up week after week until we completed this book.

- Mark Young for taking such wonderful pictures.

- Christine Clark for allowing us to photograph her doing our recommended exercises.

- Salenta Baisden, for letting us use her hands for the cover.

- Gilberto d' Urso for walking me through the art and business of publishing.

- And of course, Oprah Winfrey, who gave me a focus and inspiration to share this information with the world.

Foreword

Dear Oprah,

I just wanted to let you know I love and admire you tremendously. But I, like so many, are concerned about your health challenges. I couldn't help but notice that you've been yo-yoing back and forth on your health plan over the years. I can imagine that it can be really tough to be in the public eye where everything about your life is exposed, including your personal health battles.

My intention with this book is to help you to once again uncover that deep motivation and drive to be healthy and well, not just for now, but for the rest of your life. We want you around for a long time with all the energy and power that is Oprah.

Please use this book to take care of yourself.

Love,

Dr. Dale

Dear Reader,

This book is for you. Within all of us is an Oprah—meaning the possibility for a truly fulfilled life. But there are parts of us over which we lack mastery. If you are lacking mastery over your health, this book will help you regain it. Too often I have seen people who have lost their health, then lost their hope in their abilities to pursue their dreams. This book is about your health recovery. It is about restoring your hope. And, it is about achieving your dreams. Get ready and giddy-up!

Love,

Dr. Dale

When it comes to maintaining my health, I didn't just fall off the wagon. I let the wagon fall on me. I didn't follow my own fundamental rule of taking care of self first.

- Oprah Winfrey

Introduction

Gaining great health and longevity comes down to one thing: good decisions. Honestly, picking up this book could be one of the best decisions you've ever made for moving yourself towards a healthy you. What you do with this information is up to you, but I can tell you this, if you keep doing what you've been doing, you won't get there. To change your life, you must change!

Insanity is doing the same thing over and over again and expecting different results. – Albert Einstein.

You can't buy the trophy of great health, you have to earn it. Achieving real health will take work and that work begins with you. In the early part of this book you will find keys to motivate you to do the work necessary to getting the health results you want. Some of this work will be easy, some more challenging, but know this:

You have everything you need within you to be absolutely healthy.

Remember, health is a journey which is accomplished one step at a time. It's up to you how big a step you want to take at any given time. The key is to keep taking steps that will actually get you to health.

Unfortunately, when it comes to health, much of the information we receive is tainted by corporations or lobbyists trying to sell us something or by individuals who are misinformed. This is dangerous, because when it comes to your health, false information can kill you.

How do you know when it's good information or bad? It's all in the questions you ask. This book asks the right questions and provides correct answers. After reading this book, health will make sense for you. Here's a sample question: What are the actions and decisions I need to make that will allow my body to express health? Before the end of this book you will know the answer.

By the time you are done with this book, you will:
- Have the motivation to do what it takes to achieve optimum health
- Have discovered what is true and not true about achieving great health
- Have a workable plan you will be able to follow to get there
- Have taken steps towards practicing what you preach

All of the above will make you more powerful and more able to allow positive changes to manifest throughout your life.

Consider this book your own personal optimum health workbook – The no-BS, tell-me-like-it-is, let's get-to-it, rock and roll health transformation challenge for your life! My hope for you is that you will really enjoy the process as you progress to achieve all of your health goals.

There are many ways you can use this book. I suggest you read it through once, fill out the motivation worksheets, highlight what's important to you, underline the "aha" moments when you've discovered something that's a revelation to you, and then use it as a reference for the areas you need to work on most. This book is packed with so many revolutionary ideas and concepts that you can reread it several times, and discover new gems you may have missed before.

Enjoy!

Dr. Dale Ellwein

Purpose can be defined as: the inner drive that allows you to express who you really are and all that you can be.

Motivation: finding a strong, personal reason to move and to keep moving (no matter what).

Dr. Dale Ellwein

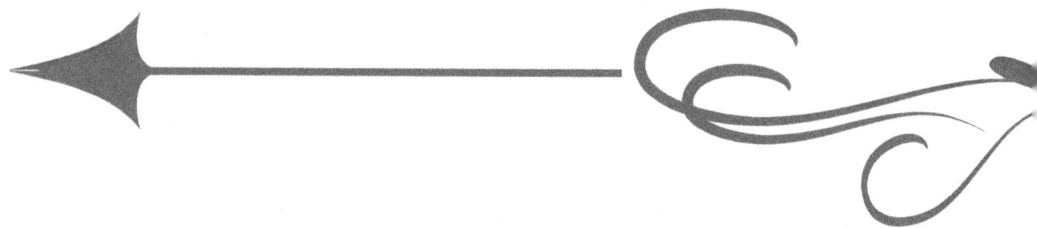

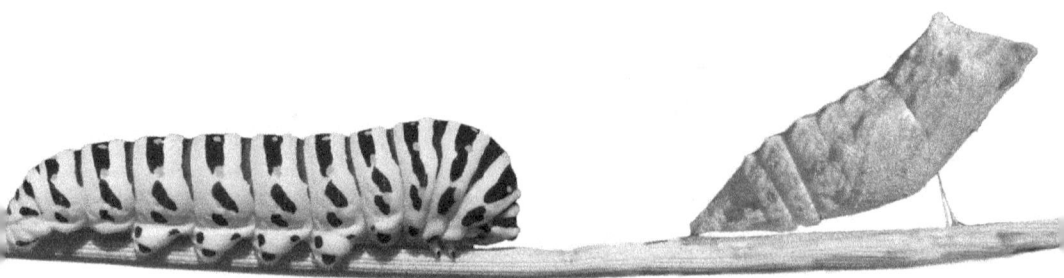

Section One
Preparing for Change

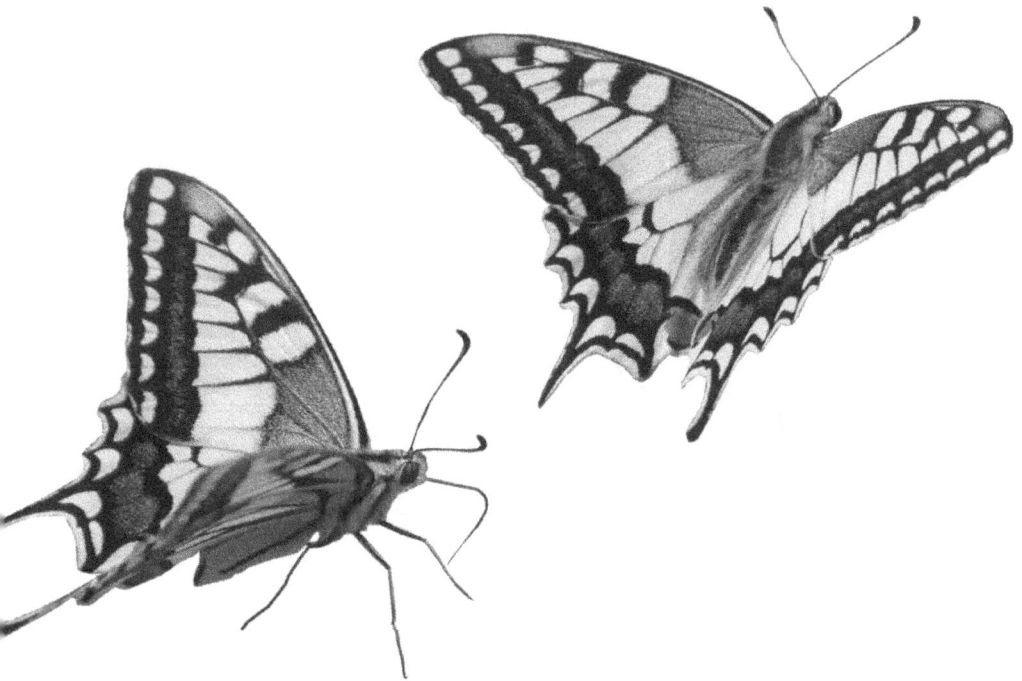

CHAPTER ONE
Motivation

*The biggest adventure you
can ever take is to live the
life of your dreams.*
- Oprah

The Key to Action

Motivation is finding a strong, personal reason to move and to keep moving towards health and longevity. People who are successful at sticking to a program for gaining great health have a strong purpose for doing so. They have great motivation. In this section I want to inspire you to make a firm and happy decision to take steps to move in the direction of health and healing as a full-time, rest-of-your-life endeavor.

The word "motivate" means to move to action.[1] Let's find out what will cause you to move and keep moving toward a long and healthy life. This will have to be a strong reason that connects to your values. It must induce you to change any bad habits that may be in the way of your achieving great health. Your motivation will also compel you to stick to your program over the long haul.

I'll give you an example from my life. I'm 46 years-old and have a very young daughter. I want to be around to see her graduate from college, to walk her down the aisle and to dance the father-daughter dance at her wedding. That might not happen for another 30 years. I'll be 76 years-old! So I want to be healthy and strong.

In addition, I don't want my children or my wife to worry about me or to have to take care of me when I grow older. I want our focus to be on personal growth and development. I want to be there for my wife and children for at least another 50 plus years, and be able to provide the means for them to truly express themselves. Without my health, I cannot provide all of us with the money, time and energy to be all that we can be as a family and as individuals.

As you see, I place a very high value on providing for my family and supporting them in every way I can. This is my strong motivator that helps me stick to my health regimens and steers me away from any habits or behavior that could compromise my good health.

1   The American Heritage® Dictionary of the English Language, Fourth Edition copyright ©2000 by Houghton Mifflin Company. Updated in 2009. Published by Houghton Mifflin Company. All rights reserved.

Here is the bottom line for me: I don't want to die early and miss all of the fun of seeing my kids grow up and miss long years of loving my wife. What's your bottom line?

The key to asking a smart, guiding question is to first pause before making the choice and taking the action. The pause allows you to get off of autopilot and take control. The pause is where new behaviors and habits begin. So, for example, what would happen if you were sitting at a table with menu in hand and you paused before deciding on your food and asked yourself this key question:

Is this food going to lead me to my health goals ...or is it going to kill me?

> **MY KEY MOTIVATION QUESTIONS**
>
> Is choosing this (food, action, thought, attitude) going to allow me to live long enough to really enjoy my life and be there for my daughter's wedding?
>
> Is this behavior going to support me into the future?

This is a great, bottom-line question. Will this help me or kill me? If you take the time to pause, you will begin to move towards establishing healthy habits.

By the way, innately, you know the answer to the above question, but our tendency is to minimize the importance of this question. Be careful. It is true that one Twinkie will not kill you today, however, a lifetime of Twinkies (and the other kinds of killing foods that someone with a Twinkie habit tends to eat) will absolutely lead to your early demise.

When it comes to exercise, if you feel too tired to go to the gym, your personal motivational question might be:

If I do the workout, will I get to my goal faster or will I just remain the slug that I have always been or that I have become?

When your questions become based on your personal values and experience, they might be quite startling. For example,

Is this food or activity or habit going to lead me to another heart attack?

Will this habit help or hinder me in making love to my spouse?

<u>Purpose</u> and <u>motivation</u> separate the successful from the unsuccessful in life. The successful have big enough reasons to do the things that other people who are not successful, don't do. Motivation, then, will allow you to shift your viewpoints, change your behavior and habits and confidently move you forward toward your goals.

How Purpose Can Get You off of Your Personal Roller Coaster

Many of us experience life as a roller coaster of ups and downs when it comes to our health. When things seem good, we experience pleasure, then we coast. (Remember, one can only coast downhill!)

Ordinarily, with many of us, when things begin to get bad, we experience pain, and then we take action. In weight loss, this is usually called yo-yoing. You hit your ideal weight and then start doing all of the bad habits that made you fat in the first place. You gain weight, get uncomfortable, and finally you begin to incorporate the good habits and drop the weight again. This is hard on the body and a very stressful way to live.

Purpose is the key to get you off of the roller coaster. If you start living your life from the point of view of purpose, you can transcend the yo-yo effect and be proactive with your health and your life.

This is worth stating again: If you start living your life from the point of view of purpose you can transcend the yo-yo effect and be proactive with your health and your life.

Again, purpose can be defined as: The inner drive that allows you to express who you really are and all that you can be.

"Weighing in at 216 pounds, the heavyweight champion of the world, Mike Tyson!" I remember this story from Tony Robbins. Sitting in the audience, Oprah was mortified when she heard these words because she realized that she weighed as much as the heavyweight champion of the world!

Too many people wait until they get hit in the face and they just can't take it anymore before they change. For some people, it's a heart attack. For others, it's the diagnosis of diabetes. For Oprah, it was weighing as much as the heavyweight champion of the world.

Once again, to get off your roller-coaster, purpose is the key. If you want to stop getting hit on the head over and over again, you need to develop a strong purpose. Yes, you may have had a wake-up call that is startling. It may have even motivated you to pick up this book, but let's work out a strategy so you don't have to keep getting hit on the head by life over and over again. A great purpose needs to address who you really are and all that you can be.

Here's one of my favorite quotes which talks about being all that you can be:

Our deepest fear is not that we are inadequate. Our deepest fear is that we are powerful beyond measure. It is our light, not our darkness, that most frightens us. We ask ourselves, Who am I to be brilliant, gorgeous, talented, fabulous? Actually, who are you not to be? You are a child of God. Your playing small does not serve the world. There is nothing enlightened about shrinking so that other people won't feel insecure around you. We are all meant to shine, as children do. We were born to make manifest the glory of God that is within us. It's not just in some of us; it's in everyone. And as we let our own light shine, we unconsciously give other people permission to do the same. As we are liberated from our own fear, our presence automatically liberates others.

Marianne Williamson

Let's uncover your purpose so you can take the steps to build the foundational habits that allow you to get off your roller coaster for good. Let's figure out what makes you shine.

Let's make it clear right now, change is uncomfortable! This isn't a book about coasting and being comfortable, there is no magic pill. How many of you know somebody who has had gastric bypass, lost a whole bunch of weight and then gained it back? The quick fix never works. You must develop strategies that will last a lifetime. We will go over these in chapter two.

Wanting to Choose Healthy Habits

Health is a choice based on decisions made moment to moment, day by day. These decisions over time become habits. Your bad habits were formed this way and now good habits can replace them in the same way. It is up to you. Before we find out what will motivate you into good health habits, let's look at what has motivated some of my clients toward health. It might give you some ideas.

Patient Motivations—some examples

A couple had become so grumpy at home the tension was building to the breaking point. The husband of this couple was considering chiropractic care with me. At the consultation the wife said, "This is cheaper than a divorce, let's write the check and do it!" That was their motivation, they were tired of the grumpy existence they had fallen into. And the result? His chiropractic program saved their marriage.

I have a Pilates instructor as a patient whose motivation is to increase her stamina and good health. She sends me her students who are motivated by the desire to excel more at both Pilates and other activities in their lives. They want to increase their endurance and skill.

I have had hairstylists whose hands had shut down and they faced the possibility of having to give up their profession because their hands didn't work anymore. With chiropractic care they were able to restore the use of their hands so they didn't have to give up their clientele or their dreams.

A man came to me for care so that he would be well enough to go through surgery and get a better result. He had gotten to the point where his body had broken down and he required surgery. At that point I couldn't help prevent the surgery, but I could help him get his body healthy enough to where he could better survive and strive through the surgery.

Cancer patients have a whole team that work to respond to their cancer and the disease process. I call this, their "defense team." When cancer patients come to me, I talk to them about the importance of having a health team as well as a sickness team. In other words, it's important to have an "offense team" as well as a "defense team" when it comes to your health. Cancer patients who come for chiropractic care are motivated by the desire for wellness and building up the body while undergoing the medical treatment of chemotherapy and radiation. Sometimes cancer survivors seek chiropractic care to help them build up their bodies after they have completed their medical treatment.

I have a songwriter who comes in for care when he gets stuck in his writing. His adjustments, he says, "Clear his neuro-net" so that he can think more clearly and create. Often times he's walking out the door of my office and he's already got his tape recorder going, talking through new ideas for songs.

People come in for care for all kinds of reasons. Whether it's a surfer who wanted to surf until he's 80 finding that at 60 he just doesn't have the stamina he needs to paddle out past a big undertow to the wave set or an artist who doesn't have the energy to get her projects done or is in too much pain to follow through. Most anyone can turn deterioration into rehabilitation with the right health program.

I've cared for new fathers; some in their 30s, 40s or 50s, who want to be able to pick up their sons or teach them to throw a football when their sons get older. I've cared for mothers who are motivated by keeping their stamina so they can do the multi-tasking required to raise a good family.

One patient of mine had an unwanted, emergency C-section with her first child and was motivated to get chiropractic care three times a week in her last trimester to enable her body to be strong enough to have a vaginal birth with her second child. As a result, with her second baby, she had only a three-hour labor and successfully, happily, gave birth vaginally at home with her midwife. She is my wife and we named the baby boy Jace.

Lots of my patients seek care to become even better at what they do— playing basketball, football, baseball or the like. We have people coming in who just want to feel better about themselves. They seek and find greater self esteem by giving themselves all the tools to help them achieve greater health.

And then we have people coming in to make the commitment because they can't take it anymore. They can no longer pick up their child, or can't eat what they want to because it gives them heartburn or some other negative consequence.

One lady patient of ours was sick five months out of the year and went to a multitude of medical doctors and specialists who couldn't figure out what was wrong with her. She came to see me and in the few weeks of her care hasn't been sick since. That was over six months ago. Further, she knows for sure that she is on the mend. This gives her great hope.

The list goes on—a woman who had daily headaches since childhood quite quickly eliminated them from her life—a tremendous relief for her and a benefit for her employer who could now expect even better work from her. A man came in who couldn't get food down until two in the afternoon because his stomach was bugging him so much. Now he can eat breakfast.

A young woman came to me with bad neck pain that she had since she was a teenager. She had been to all the big specialists and was given MRI's twice. She's now doing great as we've freed up her neck and nerve system through chiropractic care. Now she bounces in and out of my office.

One of my greatest specialties is helping musicians with hand problems. Imagine spending your whole life, committing many hours each day to become a professional musician just to have your hands give out when you begin to make it. These people call me all the time and get great results because they are motivated to have long, professional careers.

There are as many motivations as there are conditions. For example, obese patients are often motivated by the desire to do the most basic activities of daily living—tying their shoes, wiping themselves correctly or being able to walk to their cars.

In any case, motivation demands some hard work and sometimes requires that one push through a lot of effort and considerable barriers, but it's worth it.

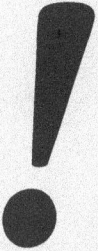

> **CAUTION:** If you find yourself saying, "I have to do such and such," know that you are coming from the position of being a victim of your goals. For instance if you say, "I have to lose weight," or "I have to eat better." A way to empower yourself is to turn this around and say, "I choose to do such and such because _____." And then find your own true reason for choosing that action. For instance, "I choose to eat better because I want to look good in my wedding dress."

"Where there is no struggle, there is no strength.
-Oprah"

Chapter Two gives you action steps to help you find motivation and purpose. Let's move on and get to it. When you hit on or evolve the right motivation and purpose for you, you will gain tremendous energy and sense of direction.

CHAPTER TWO
Action Steps for Finding Your Motivation and Purpose

Building a Lasting Purpose

Take a moment now to write down a list of the most important parts of your life.

Here is an example.

* Family
* My Work
* My Relationship with God
* My Health
* Art

Now make your list.

_____   _____

_____   _____

_____   _____

_____   _____

Prioritize the items on your list. Put a number 1 in front of the most important one, a number 2 in front of the next most important one and so on.

Look at the numbers. These are what you feel are very important to you. Awesome!

Here's the next key question.

Was your health your #1 choice? What number choice was it?

When I ask this question of my patients, in most cases health is not the number one. Here is the real question: can you really enjoy any of the other areas of your life that are important to you if your health fails? In other words, shouldn't health be your #1 priority if you want to keep enjoying all of those other areas that make up your life?

> Do the one thing that you cannot do. Fail at it. Try again. Do better the second time. The only people who never tumble are those who never mount the high wire. This is your moment, own it.
>
> – Oprah

Hopefully, this key exercise has helped you to realize the foundational importance of your health. If you want to keep doing all of the wonderful things that you enjoy and value in your life, *health must be your #1 priority.*

All you really need to do to experience optimum health long-term is to keep doing the things that get you healthy and let go of the things that prevent you from being healthy.

Let's talk about some strategies to help you get motivated and live from your purpose.

Strategies

Strategy #1: Create a Reward System

What is it you love to do but don't allow yourself to do? Is there something you'd love to have but don't allow yourself to have it? In other words what could you do or have as a reward for taking steps towards your optimum health?

For example, let's say that, as a result of this book, you and your health practitioner design a life-changing health program for you. How do you want to reward yourself for sticking to your program faithfully for a week, a month, six months, and a year? How about five years?

Do you want to reward yourself with going to a movie, or a night out with your spouse at a wonderful hotel? Is there a trip you want to take? A special person you want to go visit or meet somewhere? A play you want to see? Is there a museum you want to visit or a sporting event or concert you'd like to attend? Do you want, as a reward, to be able to buy some clothes to fit your new, slimmed-down body? Perhaps you can save some of the money you used to spend on expensive coffees, junk food and alcohol and put it towards a trip you've always wanted to take.

There has to be something in it for you to more easily stick to your new habits, so let yourself dream. You are earning the right to give these things to yourself.

A Worksheet for Designing a Reward System

Write down some ideas for how you want to reward yourself for meeting your target, hitting your goal of transformation on a weekly, monthly and yearly basis. What will you give yourself?

Here's my sample list:

Weekly:

- A pedicure or manicure
- Dinner out with my wife at her favorite restaurant

Monthly:

- A full body massage
- A facial

Yearly:

- A trip to Hawaii
- A new hot tub

Now have fun doing yours!

Weekly:

_____   _____

_____   _____

Monthly:

_____   _____

_____   _____

Yearly:

_____   _____

_____   _____

Strategy #2: Incentives (Incentive is a thing that motivates or encourages you to do something.)

I have a patient who lost 40 pounds because she wanted to go to her high school reunion and look good. Is there some place where you want to go to look good for other people?

I also have a patient who decided to run a marathon. She joined a group that practiced three times a week increasing distance and in the end, she ran the marathon.

One of my patients wanted to climb Mt. McKinley. To do this, you must reserve your space well in advance. This decision and commitment motivated him to start training in order to accomplish his goal. He got in better shape and climbed to the top of Mt. McKinley.

Write down some positive incentives that will motivate you to take action to get healthier? Please take note that incentives can be single occurrences and may not be sustainable. However, if you continue to find new incentives throughout your life, you will always have reasons to keep healthy.

_____   _____

_____   _____

_____   _____

Strategy #3: Days Off

Sometimes it is easier to stay disciplined with your eating if you know that it is a choice. The concept of never getting to eat something that you really like can be daunting. Here is a trick that works well.

Purchase a pocket notepad. (Of course, these days there may actually be an application for your iPhone or smart phone that you could use). Carry the notepad around with you as you go through your day. When you get a craving for something, write it down. Once a week, take the day off from your eating regimen and eat one item from your list in the notepad.

With this strategy, one of a few things will happen. Usually, after you write your craving in your notebook, the craving will pass. When your "day off" comes along, you won't eat everything that you have written, you will choose one thing. Finally, since your body will be changing and getting healthier, whatever you eat from your list in your book may now make you feel queasy or sick and therefore you might not want it again!

Strategy #4: Starting with Something Good for You

Health is not necessarily "all or nothing." If you do one thing healthier for yourself today, you are farther along than if you did nothing at all. In this strategy the goal is to add healthy things to your life. Dr. James Chestnut has coined the term, "Fresh Fiber First." This means, you simply eat a piece of fruit or vegetable before you eat anything else. Not only are you eating something good to start with, but also you are filling your stomach so you won't eat as much or crave bad foods as much.

Make a List of Good Things You Can Add Easily

Here are some examples: Start taking a good multiple vitamin, take fish oil in the morning, eat a salad once a day, go for a walk first thing in the day and go to a good chiropractor.

What Is Your Motivation?

This point in the chapter is where the rubber meets the road.

_____ _____

_____ _____

_____ _____

A Perception Exercise to Get You Going

1. Write down all the words that you feel describe who you are (i.e. witty, intelligent, caring, competent, skilled, etc.)
2. Look in the mirror. Write down what you see as objectively as possible.
3. How do you feel about what you see in the mirror? To what extent do your best qualities shine through your physical self?
4. Does your view of your physical self match up to your vision of non-physical self?
5. Now look in the mirror and write down all the words that describe how you imagine you are being perceived by others.
6. Take a look at all your answers above. Are they in sync or not? What do you need to do, health wise, to get your personal traits in sync with how you want to be perceived by yourself and others? Write your thoughts about these things. Can you see how this can motivate you?
7. Sketch out a plan to get how you feel about yourself in sync with how you look. What steps do you need to take to get you where you want to go? Do you need to…

- Spruce up your image? (get a new haircut, get some new clothes, hire a color consultant?)
- Lose weight, gain weight?
- Hire an organizer?
- Make changes in your house?
- Make an appointment with your chiropractor to help you with posture?
- Make an appointment with a nutritionist?
- Learn what exercise is best for your body and how often?
- Other?

Turn these answers into a checklist and get started.

Motivation Worksheet

Once you set your motivation, you will have the foundation that allows you to go forward towards a lifetime of health.

In this next exercise, here are the rules:

1. Complete each sentence.

2. Answer with the first thing that comes to your mind.

3. Repeat answers are not allowed.

4. Keep going until you exhaust all answers. (Below, there are only four lines, but you may need more. Use a separate piece of paper as needed.)

For even better results for this exercise, get a friend to ask you the questions and record the answers.

Fill in the blank.

I choose to be healthy because_____

I choose to be healthy because_____

I choose to be healthy because_____

I choose to be healthy because_____

I am worthy of love because_____

I am worthy of love because_____

I am worthy of love because_____

I am worthy of love because_____

I know I'm ready to_____

I know I'm ready to_____

I know I'm ready to_____

I know I'm ready to_____

I'm motivated by _____

I'm motivated by _____

I'm motivated by _____

I'm motivated by _____

I want to live longer because_____

I want to live longer because_____

I want to live longer because_____

I want to live longer because_____

What has stopped me is_____

What has stopped me is_____

What has stopped me is_____

What has stopped me is_____

I will no longer be stopped because _____

I will no longer be stopped because _____

I will no longer be stopped because _____

I will no longer be stopped because _____

My biggest excuse is_____

My biggest excuse is_____

My biggest excuse is_____

My biggest excuse is_____

I will stick to my health program this time because _____

I will stick to my health program this time because _____

I will stick to my health program this time because _____

I will stick to my health program this time because _____

In addition to the above, here is a very important aspect to motivation. This may surprise you because symptoms are often viewed as things to get rid of fast. But here is another viewpoint I would like you to consider.

How Symptoms Can Motivate You

The subject of symptoms is important for you to know about in motivating and monitoring your health.

Symptoms—what are they?

Symptoms are the way that your body communicates with your conscious mind. They provide wake-up calls. They say, "Hey! Wake up! Stop doing that!"

I have a daughter named Evan. When she was an infant, she had one major way of communicating. She cried. If she was hungry, she cried. If she was tired, she cried. If she was scared, she cried. If she needed to feel loved, she cried. Your body has only one way of letting you know that it needs your attention, it produces symptoms. If you don't listen, the symptoms get louder.

Your body communicates through symptoms to direct you to make changes that will allow you to be healthy again.

There are two main reasons why we get symptoms. We are not giving the body something that it needs or we are making our body toxic.

If we just numb out our symptoms, it interferes with our body's desire to save itself. I cannot imagine quieting down my daughter because she requires love and attention, but this is often what you do to your body when you drug it.

> **THE WILTING PLANT ANALOGY***
>
> If you have a wilting plant, what do you do? First you recognize the symptom—your plant is wilting! You try adding water and if that doesn't work, you try nutrients, and/or sunlight. In other words, you are asking: what is this plant lacking—what is its deficiency?
>
> Now if your plant is still wilting, you may want to make sure the cat isn't using it as a litter box! In other words, what are some toxins the plant may be receiving that you may need to remove?
>
> So if you notice some symptoms going on in your body, think of the wilting plant. Guided by your symptoms, ask yourself, what am I lacking that I need to add: either to my diet, exercise regimen or thought processes, and/or, what are some toxins that I need to eliminate from my body, mind or environment?
>
> * Chestnut, Dr. James L. The Wellness Paradigm (2011) The Wellness Practice-Global Self Help Corp (TWP Press), Victoria, B.C. Canada page 57.

What will continue to motivate you is that your body will start to speak to you again in the form of symptoms. Not only that, but you will listen and take action instead of "living with it," because you say "that's normal for me." Many who abuse their bodies with bad health habits no longer are able to "hear" the symptoms in their bodies. They have been so self-abusive with their habits for years and years that they cannot hear their bodies when things are going wrong until they reach some kind of crisis—at which point the body screams at them. For example, a person has a heart attack. He can no longer ignore the symptoms, his body has shouted at him and he is now forced to listen.

This kind of "motivation" is dangerous. We urge you to listen to your body now, get in tune with it, by getting it healthy enough to communicate with you again.

Reminder: You can't buy a trophy for achieving good health, you have to earn it. Let's see how you can earn your trophy in the following chapters.

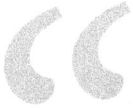

Ultimately it is your choices and actions that determine which way you are moving at any given time: toward health or toward sickness and death. Meaning, you have total responsibility over how healthy you want to be.

– Dr. Dale Ellwein

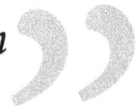

CHAPTER THREE
Truth & Lies About Health

World Health Organization's Definition of Health

Health is a state of complete physical, mental and social well being—not merely the absence of disease and infirmities.

Listening To Your Body

When I ask people, "What is Health," the most common answer I get is, "When I feel good." As we just learned in the previous chapter, health is not a lack of symptoms. In fact, often the symptoms are the cure.

You need to learn to understand your symptoms rather than to quiet them, ignore them or to shut them down. Often our symptoms guide and direct us to make more positive lifestyle changes.

Four Big Lies That Are Holding Your Health Hostage

What if something you thought to be true turned out to be false? How soon would you want to know what the real truth is? As you read forward into this section, you might be amazed at the crazy stuff we buy

Examples of How Symptoms Are the Cure

1. Let's say you eat something that's bad for you. What does your healthy body automatically do? Your body will want to get rid of it as soon as possible. Because if it doesn't, that something bad that you ate could kill you. So your body makes you vomit, and have very intense diarrhea. This is one example of how symptoms are the cure.

2. You catch a bug—for example, a bacterial infection. One of the things your body is going to do is give you a fever. In chemistry, if you want to accelerate a chemical reaction, you heat it up. The same thing is happening with your body. By heating it up, it allows your immune system to work faster. So not all fevers are something to immediately eradicate. This is another way a symptom is a cure.

into that is just not true. You may even get upset, because while it's correct that truth sets you free, it can also make you miserable at first!

Think about it, in just a few minutes, you will know the four biggest lies that are holding your health hostage! So let's get to it.

Big Lie #1: No symptoms equals good health.

Lack of symptoms does not guarantee one has good health. There are many people who have dropped dead even when they felt great. For example, Sergei Grinkov, a Russian figure skater who, together with partner (and wife) Ekaterina Gordeeva, was the 1988 and 1994 Olympic Champion and four-time World Champion.

At the age of 28, he suffered a heart attack and died.

Bob Young, the executive director of the International Skating Center said, "I'd never seen anyone in better condition. Never. I'd put him up against any athlete in any sport. I never even knew him to be sick."

Often, people go in for a regular check-up and find that they have high blood pressure, diabetes, high cholesterol, or even cancer. Before diagnosis, they felt fine and had no idea that they were unhealthy.

The Truth:

How you feel is not a good gauge of how healthy you are.

Big Lie #2: Your genes are totally responsible for your health.

Let me explain. Several years ago you may remember being taught in science class that 75% of all diseases are genetically based. In other words, if you are fat, it is because you were born with the fat gene, if you have breast cancer, you must have the breast cancer gene, if you have heart disease, you must have the heart disease gene and so on. Now, a recent Harvard study says it's 25%. I am sure that eventually it will be down to 3% or less. This is why.

When you look at genes and study them, you will find that they have not changed much in 20,000 years. That's a long time. In genetic science circles, this is no longer debated, it is just understood. Here is the first key question: "Were there obese hunter-gatherers 20,000 years ago?" When you look at present day hunter-gatherer tribes, they have the physiques of world-class athletes. What would have happened if the hunter-gatherer was obese 20,000 years ago? Might they have been eaten because they couldn't run fast? Did the hunter-gatherer have breast cancer? No! Did they develop heart disease? No! In fact, later on in the book you will find out where these diseases come from, and they are not from your genes.

You may be thinking, "Well, hunter-gatherers did not live that long, not as long as we do today." This is true. Most hunter gatherers died from trauma at an early age. They died young because they were trying to kill bison and bear with sticks and stones. It was a very dangerous time for the young warrior. However, once they became elders, they lived a long, healthy life. They sent the young ones out to hunt.

According to James L. Chestnut in his lectures and book *The Innate Diet and Natural Health*, page 38, he references an article in *The European Journal of Clinical Nutrition* (1997: 51; 207-216) by Eaton, Eaton and Konner, "Members of technologically primitive cultures who survive to the age of 60 years or more, remain relatively free from these disorders (coronary heart disease, hypertension, diabetes and some types of cancer), unlike their 'civilized' counterparts."

The Truth:

The truth is, you do not get sick because of your genes. Genetically, you are still a hunter-gatherer. Even if your mother had cancer and your sister had cancer, it does not mean that you will have cancer. Even if your grandfather and father died of heart attacks, it does not mean that you will die of a heart attack.

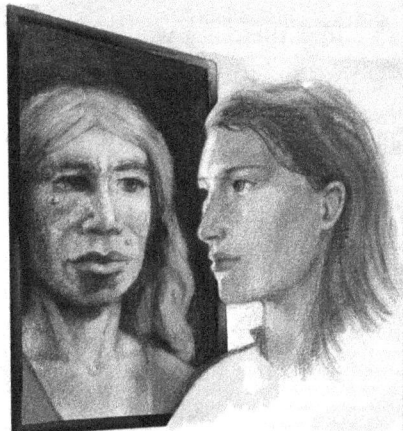

We are Hunter-Gatherers living in a modern society

There is such a thing as genetic predisposition. What this means is you may have something like breast cancer running in your family. How I describe this to my patients is that we all have weak links in our genetic chain. Like all chains, the weak links will not pop unless you stress them.

As you read this book, you will come to understand that your genes are quite perfect as long as they are not stressed to the point of failure. They are responding to your environment to either produce a state of health and healing in your body or a state of survival to overcome threats to your well being.

Genes
How Your Genes Are Perfect

Genes are designed to produce everything that your body needs—on demand—for your survival and your health. They are an amazing part of the amazing you. In order to understand your genes, we have to understand where you've come from, because your body operates in the same way as bodies did 20,000 years ago. Our bodies have not changed, but what about our societies? The changes in our societies are the culprits in all of our major health challenges and a big reason why I wrote this book. I need to help people address these changes and get back to basics.

> "Genetically our bodies are virtually the same as they were at the end of the Paleolithic era some 20,000 years ago. The appearance of agriculture and domestication of animals some 10,000 years ago and the industrial revolution some 200 years ago introduced new dietary pressures for which no adaptation has been possible in such a short time span. Thus an inevitable discordance exists between our dietary intake and what our genes are suited to."

Mann, NJ. 2004 Paleolithic Nutrition: What can we learn from the past? Asia Pac J Clin Nutr: 13 (Suppl): S17

Who Profits from Big Lie #2?

Today there is a whole industry studying genes to find the next new breakthrough drug to heal humankind. This is <u>big</u> business. They have discovered all kinds of genes that they say are responsible for the woes of our civilization. As Dr. James Chestnut says, "They even discovered a hangover gene. I know I've got it because when I drink, I get a hangover! You know what? When I don't drink, I don't get a hangover."

Do you see the fallacy in this reasoning, the flaw in relying on gene therapy? It is the outside influence of the alcohol (your lifestyle choice) that triggers the gene that leads to the hangover. Wouldn't it make better sense to choose a better lifestyle and let your perfect genes be?

The scary part about relying on genes as a determinant of your health is seen in the example of the breast cancer gene. Many women are being convinced to lop off a breast based on their genes. In other words, if a woman's sister and mother had breast cancer, she is often being convinced to take off her breast(s) as a preventative measure. It is sad and it angers me. Sure, the doctors who advise this think that they are doing what's best. However, with what you now know about genes, do you still think it is a good idea? Is it the genes or is it the environmental choices? I remember Dr. Chestnut saying something like … I can tell you one thing, if it was the testicular cancer gene that they were selling, no man would be lining up to get his boys cut off!

Your genes are followers. They do what they are told based on the signals that your body gives them. These signals are determined by your lifestyle choices: how you eat and move and how you think. You just received a preview of what's to come. For now, let's just say that in order to study your stress and your health, we must compare the environment and lifestyle of your ancestors to your environment and lifestyle now. With this new perspective, you will have the tools necessary to live a healthy 120 years.

Big Lie #3: You're sick because you are unlucky.

I remember paging through a Merck Manual while I was in chiropractic school. You know, this is the book that contains every disease known to man. I discovered in reading this medical "bible," there were rarely any causes of diseases known in medicine. In the book, written after a very high percentage of the diseases, is the word "idiopathic" which means "from an obscure or unknown cause." Isaac Asimov called idiopathic, "A high-flown term to conceal ignorance." In the television show, House, the lead character remarks that the word "comes from the Latin, meaning 'we're idiots, because we don't know what's causing it.'"

The Truth:

You do not get sick because you are unlucky. Just because they don't know what caused a disease does not mean that you are just unlucky.

Have you noticed? Most of these big lies, if they were true, would totally dis-empower you when it comes to your health. In other words, "You are just born that way," "You are unlucky," "I'm sorry, it's just the way it is," or "Don't worry, we're developing a magic pill for you."

Big Lie #4: Don't worry, we are developing a magic pill.

Do you really believe that there will be a magic pill? How many years have they been looking for the cure for cancer? Did you know that the big solution they have for cancer right now is early detection? This is part of the defense used by medical treatment, not the offense of living a better lifestyle and being proactive about steps to health and healing so that you can prevent cancer, or if you do develop it, have a better chance of survival.

Let me explain this further. When you look at medical statistics, they are now detecting cancer around two years earlier than they used to. In fact, five-year survival rate for cancer has improved dramatically. But mortality rates have not changed. According to an article from the Journal of the American Medical Association titled Are Increasing 5 –year Survival Rates Evidence of Success Against Cancer? medical doctors, Welch, Schwartz and Woloshin conclude, "Although five-year survival is a valid measure for comparing cancer therapies in a randomized trial, our analysis shows that changes in five-year survival over time bear little relationship to changes in cancer mortality. Instead, they appear primarily related to changing patterns of diagnosis."[2]

So yes, they discover it earlier and treat you with chemotherapy and radiation for a longer period of time before you die. However, people are still living generally the same amount of time. Please understand that I know there are a lot of cancer survivors out there that may be put off by these statements. Read on and you will understand that the focus of this discussion is to empower you and your upcoming generations so that they are not made victims of these lies.

The Truth:

There is no magic pill. There never will be.

Those are four of the biggest lies that are holding your health hostage. Did you notice what they have in common? Let's take a look at them right now.
1. The goal of health is ridding the body of symptoms.
2. You're sick because of your genes.
3. You're sick because you are unlucky.
4. There will be a magic pill that will take care of everything.

If you were to believe these statements, then you have absolutely no power over your own health.

Your health is in someone else's hands and that is the biggest lie of all.

2   JAMA, June14, 2000—Vol 283, No 22

CHAPTER FOUR
The Health Continuum, What's Stress Got To Do With It?

How healthy are you? Let me introduce to you the Health Continuum. I first learned of this from Patrick Gentempo who developed the "Creating Wellness Program." (See *www.creatingwellness.com* for more information.)

Continuum means a range of points on a scale from one end to another. For instance, when you sit at a piano you have a continuum from the base keys on the left all the way to the treble keys on the right. A health continuum is a scale that ranges from death and disease to optimum health and living.

The Health Continuum

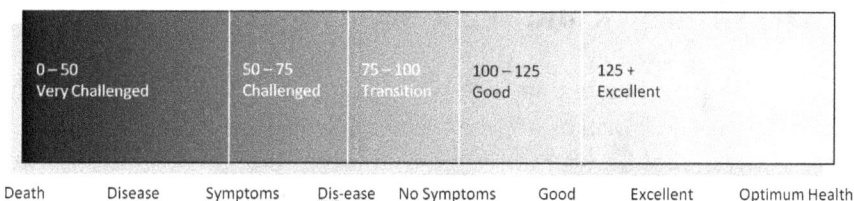

0 – 50 Very Challenged	50 – 75 Challenged	75 – 100 Transition	100 – 125 Good	125 + Excellent

Death	Disease	Symptoms	Dis-ease	No Symptoms	Good	Excellent	Optimum Health

Health and sickness exist on the same continuum. As you follow the continuum from left to right, it goes from death, to disease, to symptoms, to dis-ease, to average health (at about 100), to good health, to excellent health, to optimum health. Your level of health exists somewhere on this continuum. The thing is, you are always moving on this continuum, it is never static. You are either moving from sickness and disease, towards health and healing, or you are moving away from health and healing towards sickness and disease. In which direction are <u>you</u> moving?

The good news is that you can move towards health and healing at any time. Our bodies always want to move towards health and healing, so it is your natural tendency to do so. For example, if a person stops smoking, instantly the cells of the lungs start to regenerate if the damage isn't too great. You can move to the right of this scale.

Let's look at what the scale means. Notice that this scale goes from 0 at the left to 200 at the right. As I wrote above, average health exists right around 100. At 100, your biological age equals your chronological age.

- Your **biological age** is the same as your youthfulness. Have you known someone in their sixties who looks and acts and functions like they are in their forties? In this case their biological age is much less than their chronological age. In other words, this is something you can change.
- Your **chronological age** is the number of years you have been alive. Obviously, this is something you cannot change.

As you move to the left of the continuum into dis-ease, your biological age increases compared to your chronological age. You age faster. As you move to the right of the continuum, your biological age decreases compared to your chronological age. You age slower. In fact, as you move towards health and healing, you are slowing, stopping or reversing the effects of aging, as well as restoring your health. This is really the fountain of youth!

What Moves You to the Left of the Scale; What Makes You Sick and What Accelerates Your Aging?

Three questions, one answer: **Sustained Stress.** But it is not the fault of stress. A good form of stress is called challenge and most people thrive on it. Stress allowed your ancestors to survive. It allows you to survive. In fact, it is your survival mechanism. Without it you would die. So, why does stress kill you?

Stress is nothing more that the turning on of your fight or flight system. This is the system responsible for amping up your body's physiology for your survival. It prepares you, nearly instantaneously, for fighting or running away to safety so you can survive a dangerous situation. Without this fight or flight system, our ancestors would have fallen easy prey to any lion, tiger or bear that crossed their path. Oh my!

Your fight or flight system is so important, that it takes all priority over your health and regeneration systems. Do you remember *Star Trek*? When the *Enterprise* was under attack and the shields were failing, Captain James T. Kirk would transfer all power from life support to the shields. Why? Being without life support would mean death over time, but being without shields in battle would mean death right now. This is exactly what your body does. When you sense that you are under attack, your nerve system shuts down health and healing and all energy shifts to survival.

Your fight or flight system is meant to be used in short durations. You are sacrificing your health and longevity, your life support systems, to run it. You get into trouble when you run your fight or flight system for an extended period of time. When your life support system shuts down and you are running at full speed, you develop disease and die sooner than you should. In other words, you are traveling to the left of your health continuum.

What Happens to Your Body When You Are Under Stress? – The Physiology of Stress

Your cells can be in one of two states: adaptation or rejuvenation. Stress puts your cells into a state of adaptive physiology (survival mode). We would all prefer to be in rejuvenation all of the time, but when we need to survive, our bodies sacrifice rejuvenation in order for us to escape immediate danger.

> *You cannot be in growth and defense at the same time. In other words, cells cannot simultaneously move forward and backward.*
>
> **– Bruce Lipton, Ph.D.,**
> *The Biology of Belief*

To illustrate the way that our stress response is supposed to work, let's take as an example from an ancestor of ours from hunter-gatherer times.

The hunter-gatherer walks with her children down a deer trail to pick some berries. It is a lovely site and everything is wonderful until a mother bear walks around the corner with her cubs. What happens in this woman's body?

The very first thing that happens is that her nervous system detects something in her environment that could be a danger to her children and herself: the bear. The nerve system recognizes a stressor. Automatically and immediately, this puts her body into **fight-or-flight.**

Her brain sends signals down her spine to the sympathetic nerve system located in her mid-back. Her sympathetic nerve system then relays this signal to her heart, adrenal glands (stress glands), diaphragm, blood system, eyes, and everywhere else that is needed for surviving the threat. Immediately her heart rate increases, respiration increases and becomes deep, then blood pressure increases, and the blood flow to her arms and legs increases while her digestive system, immune system, reproduction systems, and many of her organs are slowed down.

Anything of your body functions that promote growth and repair are slowed down as your body amps up to allow you to survive the threat.

This may seem like a bad thing, but this is to get her out of immediate danger and it is supposed to be very short term. It's just like Captain Kirk when he's under attack and his shields are failing—he sacrifices life support in order to survive.

This exact same process happens to you in the fight or flight mode. Once again, the only reason that you have a fight or flight response is so that you can survive to get into a safe, more hospitable, nurturing environment.

Also, the **adrenal glands** (your major stress glands) are fired through the sympathetic nerve system.

The following is from my notes from the Certified Chiropractic Wellness Professional classes taught by Dr. James L. Chestnut. He used his books, The 14 Foundational Premises ™ for the Scientific and Philosophical Validation of the Chiropractic Wellness Paradigm (pgs. 16-21) and Wellness and Prevention Paradigm (pgs. 138-142) in teaching the class:

Substances Released From the Adrenal Glands

Norepinephrine, epinephrine, adrenaline, noradrenaline (catecholamines)

- Liberate free fatty acids into your blood stream for energy.
- Turn down insulin receptors so as to keep sugar in the blood stream for immediate use.
- Stimulate the release of clotting agents that are put into the blood stream in case of injuries that cause bleeding.

Cortisol

- Turns down uptake of LDL (considered "bad" cholesterol) in the liver, thus leaving more LDL in the blood system. (LDL is important for wound clotting.)
- Turns down production of HDL (considered "good" cholesterol) thus leaving less HDL in the blood.
- Breaks down glycogen to increase blood sugar.
- Breaks down protein for more blood sugar.
- Turns down the immune system (white blood cells do not save you from tigers and the immune system takes an incredible amount of energy).
- Turns down sex hormones.

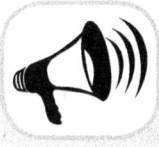

Special note: noradrenaline is also produced and released in your brain during a flight-or-flight response. What this does is heighten sensory acuity. In other words, it sharpens your senses (and sensitivity to pain). However, it also shuts down the areas of your brain for short-term memory and learning, because these areas are not needed for fight or flight. So, stress sharpens your signal detection system at the expense of concentration. This may lead to such conditions as chronic fatigue, fibromyalgia, ADD, ADHD and others.

Chronically under stress, the modern-day hunter-gatherer, you, develops fat in the belly, hips and thighs. Fat in these areas does not interfere with your ability to move around.

Also, under stress, you will crave sugar and fat. These are fuel. Back in the day of the hunter-gatherer when he craved sugar and fat he would eat a wildebeest or a mammoth or nuts and seeds for fat, and fruit for sugar. Today, you get trans fatty acids and refined sugars. These increase blood sugar even more, which increases insulin, and makes you fatter faster.

In summary, when we look at all of the adaptive physiology that comes from fight-or-flight, we can see that it is a natural, good thing in the short term. It is designed to get us out of trouble. However, in today's modern society, we live in fight or flight most of the time. This leads to all of the chronic illnesses of our times.

A Closer Look at Stress

There are four phases of stress as outlined by Hans Selye, Hungarian endocrinologist. These are the stages that your body goes through as it continues to be stressed. They are:

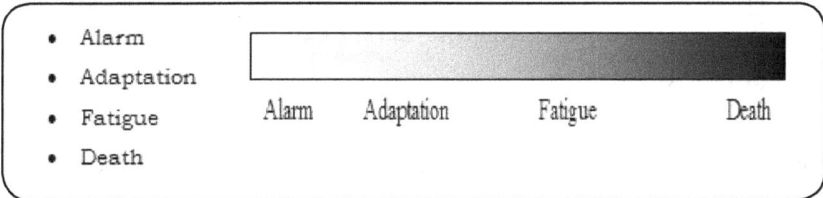

- Alarm
- Adaptation
- Fatigue
- Death

Alarm   Adaptation   Fatigue   Death

Alarm

The alarm stage is the initial reaction to a stressor. It is the automatic switching on of your fight or flight system and the turning down of your regenerative, healing system. When the alarm goes off, you are ready to fight or run. It's survival time!

Steven Spielberg is a master at triggering alarm in his audience. Do you remember *Jaws*? Richard Dreyfus's character is investigating an abandoned sailboat. He dives under the boat and with his flashlight he sees a hole in the bottom of the boat. Stuck in the wood of the hole is a giant shark tooth. He pries at it with his knife. He hits it and works at it. The music starts, du dud, du dud, du du du du du du du dud. He hits it one more time. Suddenly, a waterlogged head falls into the hole! Instant alarm. Everyone in the audience jumps. A whole generation might never feel comfortable in the ocean again.

Some people get stuck in this stage of stress. They tend to be very jumpy, stressed out, nervous, highly reactive and volatile. They constantly are under the expectation that something is going to get them.

Healthy individuals go into the alarm stage of stress and after the situation has been handled, go back into health and regeneration.

An example of a healthy reaction is seen on the plains of Africa every day. Imagine a zebra grazing on the plains. Suddenly a lion is charging and the chase is on. The zebra is in total alarm mode as it dashes left and right to avoid the lion's deadly claws. Suddenly, the lion gives up and the zebra gallops away. The zebra, realizing that it got away and that the stressor is gone, takes a deep breath, lets it out and thinks, "Whew, that was close. Hey, there's some grass over there." And then it goes over and grazes.

Adaptation

The adaptation phase of your stress response has to do with taking action. First, the alarm triggers and it is time to move. This is adaptation. Adaptation usually involves getting you to a safe place so that you can return to health and regeneration. There are two kinds of adaptation. One is positive and the other is negative. Let me explain.

Positive Adaptation

Let's say that you begin to exercise. In order to build muscle or stamina, you must put a load on your system. In muscle building, this means that you lift more than you usually do. You stress your body and your body adapts by growing your muscles. In building stamina, you run a little more than usual. This puts stress on your body and you adapt and build stamina. This is positive adaptation.

Negative Adaptation—Sometimes Known as Chronic Adaptive Physiology (dis-ease)

Chronic Adaptive Physiology is just another way of saying that a person is in a state of fight or flight all the time. So, let's say that you get stuck in adaptation. The alarm has gone off and the stress is always on. Your body is trying to get you to change your environment and get to safety, but you are not moving. Your body perceives that it is always in danger. **What does your body do to make you take action to get you to safety? It creates symptoms.**

If you are under constant stress, what happens to your body chemistry (also known as physiology)? Your heart rate increases, your blood pressure goes up, your LDL cholesterol goes up, your digestive system slows, your sex hormones diminish, your concentration falters. Your immune system drops. You're stressed!

So how does this look to you? Over time, you develop heart palpitations, upset stomach, indigestion, colitis, stomach ulcers, headaches, body pains, angina, blood clots, infertility, irritability, high blood pressure, loss of concentration, depression, etc. This is your body saying to you, "Come on! We have got to get you out of this life or death situation!"

Fatigue

The fatigue phase is where you really become "sick." This is when you have been in stress for so long that you are broken down to the point where you are most likely to be labeled with a disease. Medical intervention may be required at this time. In this phase many have heart attacks, cancer, emphysema, type II diabetes, obesity, arthritis and so on.

A slang expression for the fatigue phase is "one foot in the grave." There are whole rest homes filled with people in the fatigue phase of stress. Most medical doctors say that diseases created by prolonged stress are just part of getting old. With what you already know about stress, you can see the flaw in this view. The major diseases of "civilized" societies are caused by prolonged stress!

In today's modern society, we live in fight or flight most of the time—chronic adaptive physiology—and this leads to all of the chronic illnesses of our times. Take a look at some of the naturally occurring fight or flight responses that occur when you are stressed and what happens in the following diseases.

As you read this, notice how all of the "symptoms" that lead to and define these diseases are good when running away from a lion. Where we get into trouble is when we keep these systems running at this level through fatigue.

The following is from my notes from the Certified Chiropractic Wellness Professional classes taught by Dr. James L. Chestnut and from his book *The 14 Foundational Premises ™ for the Scientific and Philosophical Validation of the Chiropractic Wellness Paradigm* (pgs. 20-23).

Heart Disease and Stroke

- Increased platelets and clotting factors (good when bitten by a lion)
- Increased blood pressure and heart rate (good to get blood and nutrients circulating in your body.)
- Increased LDL and lower HDL (good, see box below)

Which is the "bad" cholesterol?

Drug companies would have you believe that your LDL cholesterol is bad. LDL cholesterol is very important if you are in "fight or flight" for two reasons:

LDL cholesterol is a clotting factor. If you were bitten by a lion, you want to have a lot of that around or you'll bleed to death.

LDL is a precursor to your stress hormones. This means, LDL can be easily converted into a stress hormone. If you are burning up your stress hormones, you want a lot of this in reserve.

Diabetes

- Increased blood sugar and insulin resistance (good because blood sugar is your rocket fuel that you burn in order to escape the lion)

Cancer (breast, prostate, ovary, testicular cancers)

- Turned down immune system (good because you devote that energy to escape the lion)
- Turned down sex hormones (not needed when running away from a lion)
- Chronic increased insulin (good because it allows blood sugar to remain in the blood stream to be used as needed)

ADHD, Fibromyalgia, Chronic Fatigue

- Heightened sensory reception (got to know where the lion is and the escape routes!)

- Decreased ability to focus, concentrate and memorize (not needed when running away from a lion)

All Digestive Problems

- Shunting blood and energy from the digestive tract to the arms and legs (good when running from the lion, digestion takes energy that is better used in the escape process)

In Summary: The major health challenges today that create early death and poor quality of life are little more than your stress response running for way too long. The greatest thing about this information is that you determine your health by addressing the causes of your stress and adopting a lifestyle that supports your health and your perfect genes.

The bottom line is this: the things you need in order to get away from (a lion) are amped up, the things you don't need are shut down. But we don't want to live, day by day as if we are being chased by a lion.

Thank you again, Dr. Chestnut, for the above information.

The Deadly Aspect of Drugs

As I wrote earlier, symptoms can be the cure, or at least, lead to the cure. But, instead of listening to what the symptoms mean, changing one's lifestyle and getting to a practitioner who can get to the cause of the problem, what do most people do? The usual response is to ignore them until they get so bad that one rushes to a medical doctor who will help them cover up the symptoms with drugs. Now that you know more about stress and symptoms, can you see how this is not necessarily a good idea?

Masking symptoms with drugs may create a change in the symptoms, however it does not get rid of the stress response. Take the cholesterol medication, Lipitor. I remember when the drug first came out. The commercial said that Lipitor has been shown to lower cholesterol *with diet and exercise*, and Lipitor may not reduce your risk of heart attack. Now you know why. Lipitor does nothing for your stress response that is still affecting your entire body. The drug may reduce your LDL cholesterol levels. However, your body wants to increase the LDL cholesterol in order to respond to the stressor. LDL and all of the stress responses are good things if you are trying to survive short term. Most drugs are tested short term (weeks). They don't tell you that, yes, your cholesterol will be lower, but you'll most likely die earlier.

Let's look at blood pressure medicines. If you are stuck in the adaptive phase of stress, often your blood pressure elevates. When you go to the medical doctor, they give you a drug to lower your blood pressure. You take it and it goes down. What does your body do? It's still under stress and thinks that you are still in a life or death situation. Your body reads that your blood pressure is low and tries to raise it, but it can't. This accelerates you to the fatigue stage of stress.

Let's say that you want to quit the drug. You stop and your blood pressure shoots up. Why? Because your body is pushing for it to go up and when the drug is removed, it shoots up. It's like when you kink a hose. Pressure builds, but the kink (the drug) keeps it from flowing. When you un-kink the hose (stop the drug), the water squirts out. Of course the doctor says, "See. You still have high blood pressure. You need to go back on the meds."

Death

The final phase of prolonged stress is death. Like anything that runs too long, wearing and tearing down the machinery, death occurs. Remember, there are two systems running your body, rejuvenation and survival. Those who live in survival for most of their lives will die earlier.

I know that this has been a big bite of information, but your health depends on your knowing the truth of where diseases originate. With this understanding, we can work to develop a perfect program to help move you out of fight-or-flight and into health and healing.

How Do You Spot Where You Are on the Scale?

Ask yourself, "Where am I on this scale today?" Make an "X" where you believe your health is on the continuum.

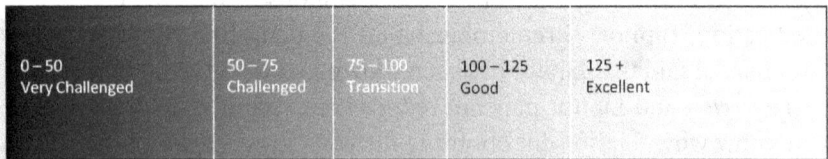

0 – 50 Very Challenged	50 – 75 Challenged	75 – 100 Transition	100 – 125 Good	125 + Excellent

Death	Disease	Symptoms	Dis-ease	No Symptoms	Good	Excellent	Optimum Health

Now, make an "X" where you would like to be. Now you have a goal and you can re-assess yourself on a regular basis to see how you think you are doing. See Appendix #4 for a more scientific way to find out where you are on the health continuum.

Remember, Life Does Not Stand Still

Every decision you make moves you either toward wellness or toward sickness on the health continuum. Remember, it is the decisions you consistently make that become your habits and your habits become your overall lifestyle. In what direction are you moving?

How Do You Move To the Right of the Scale?

The magic question! In a nutshell, the way to move to the right of the scale is to decrease your stress load and/or increase your capacity to handle stress. There are four major ingredients to address in order to create your perfect health. You could also say you have to develop good habits in each of the following:

- The Way You Eat and What You Take into the Body
- The Way You Move
- The Way You Think
- The Way You Take Care of Your Nerve System

We will address these four elements for you in Section Two: Moving Towards Optimum Health.

In the next chapter you will learn the differences between medical and alternative care and when to use each. Then, you will be given the Health Formula and invited to make a written commitment to your health betterment program.

CHAPTER FIVE
The Health Formula and Your Commitment

Choosing the Right Form of Health Practice

Nobody's journey is seamless or smooth. We all stumble. We all have setbacks. It's just life's way of saying, "Time to change course." – Oprah

The Traditional Medical Approach As Opposed to the Alternative Health Approach

Here is the first thing that I want to be clear about—in a crisis, an emergency situation, there is nothing better than traditional medical care. If I break my arm in an accident, I am not running to the chiropractor or any other "alternative" health practitioner first. I'm going to the emergency room or the medical doctor's office ASAP!

Now when it comes to health, in the absence of a crisis emergency situation, the first thing most traditional medical doctors do is to measure your symptoms and determine if they can label them as a disease or syndrome. Remember, most symptoms you are seeking to resolve are the result of your chronic state of "fight-or-flight."

Once they have a label for your symptoms, their goal is to shut them off so that you cannot feel them. They usually do this with drugs and when the drugs no longer work or your condition worsens, they use surgery. By the way, in a vast majority of the diseases that they can label you with, they say the cause is unknown. As I mentioned earlier, the fancy word for this is "idiopathic." Now that you understand "fight or flight," you now know where most diseases originate.

The majority of medical doctors do not engage in finding out what lifestyle changes need to occur to resolve the situation that resulted in the symptoms. In effect, the conventional medical doctor says, "Let's do our best to shut the symptoms down to make you comfortable and so you don't have to change a thing in your life."

The "alternative" health practitioner works to get to the bottom of your symptoms; examining the habits or stressors that are creating the symptoms that cause your suffering. In other words, they not only look and listen to your body but also probe and explore your lifestyle to isolate the factors in your life that are not supporting your health. These factors are always something the patient can change, and with understanding and discipline, control. Also, in most cases, this doctor teaches and empowers you to read your body symptoms and change your behaviors according to what the symptoms are telling you. In other words, you learn to listen to your body.

The Chili Dog Analogy

Let's say you love chili dogs. You eat three of them and your stomach hurts! You go to the medical doctor. The med doctor says, "Take this antacid," and you feel better. You keep eating chili dogs and taking your antacid. Eventually your stomach develops an ulcer. You go to the medical doctor, they run thousands of dollars of tests, they tell you have an ulcer and they give you a drug. You keep eating chili dogs. The drug stops working and your stomach starts bugging you again. You go to the medical doctor who runs even more impressive, expensive tests and tells you you've got stomach cancer. They give you chemo and radiation and hopefully you survive. You keep eating chili dogs.

Chili Dogs, the Alternative

You love chili dogs. You eat three of them and your stomach hurts! You go to an "alternative" health practitioner. He or she asks, "What were you eating?" You say "Three chili dogs." The practitioner suggests you reduce or stop your chili dog intake! You stop, you feel better, problem solved. No drugs, no expensive tests, no surgery, no cancer.

The Health Formula

The Health Formula is: Your Environment + Your Genetic Response to Your Environment = Your Physiology

By environment I mean your choices that make up your lifestyle, the world you live in, the people surrounding you.

Genetic response is the pre-programmed reaction to the environment based on eons of experience passed down from generation to generation via the genes. As an example; if you live at sea level and move to Denver (the mile high city) your genes will respond to the lack of oxygen by creating more red blood cells.

Your physiology is your internal bio-chemical expression of health or dis-ease.

This is how the health formula is seen to work. Your environment (Denver) has less oxygen than you're used to. Your body responds (genetic response) by making more red blood cells (your new physiology) This adaptation allows you to have better health than when you first arrived in Denver.

Rejuvenation is defined as building, rebuilding and restoring. You could say it is the restoring of the youthful appearance of something. (The word comes from the Latin *Juvenis* meaning "a youth.")

Adaptation is about reacting to the environment so that one can survive. Rejuvenation is about rebuilding your body, restoring it, or moving it towards what was ideal in youth. That isn't cosmetic so much as it is interior health—making the organs and all systems of the body work to their optimum efficiency.

Bodies do wear out. But one can rebuild and restore the body towards a youthful ideal. In fact, some 20 year-olds lead such a damaging lifestyle, their bodies can "age" too quickly and they can look older than a healthy, fit 60 year-old.

One has to know what habits to change and which new ones to adopt.

As a society, you see people doing the same thing over and over expecting different results all the time. For instance, if I'm an investor and I'm just playing the numbers from the point of view of fear about what's going on in the economy so much that I decide to just sell everything, that is reacting to the environment. Whereas, really good investors will say, "We'll see. And we'll hold on and ride it out. And when it does drop all the way down to the bottom, we'll buy more and then ride it back up." The scared investors are too afraid and too busy reacting to what's going on in the marketplace.

> *Insanity is doing the same thing over and over again and expecting different results.*
>
> – **Albert Einstein**

When it comes to our health, a lot of us are reactive. We start to feel tired, we drink some coffee or an energy drink. We feel better temporarily, but later feel even more tired. We have another energy drink. We feel awful a few hours later. An individual cannot keep doing the same thing over and over again in health and expect a different result. We have to get to the bottom of why we are tired.

Let's say you are in "fight or flight" and your physiology is trying to get you out of danger by raising your blood pressure. If you take a pill to try to lower it, it is not going to produce health because the environmental stressor is still there and your body is still in "fight or flight." Your body reads that your blood pressure is artificially lowered and because it is in "flight or flight" it puts out even more stress hormones in the attempt to raise your blood pressure for your survival. The increased stress hormones can potentially create other effects, known as side effects. Then, you go back to the doctor to get another pill to control the latest side effect which causes your body to put out more stress hormones and it keeps going on and on like this. That is doing the same thing over and over again and expecting a different result.

This book has been outlining the route to vibrant health and energy. In order to be healthy, you need to do all of the key steps, there are no short cuts. It takes knowledge, great choices and orderly progress in a consistent way towards the goal of optimum health.

Now, can you be healthy and not fit? Probably not. Always aim to be healthy *and* fit.

Make It a Must!

Have you ever wanted to do something and then didn't? It almost feels like a silly question, doesn't it?

We all have things that we know that we should do or even need to do, but we don't. Why? This little question is the biggest problem. When we start asking ourselves, "Why am I not doing this?" or, "Why did I do that?" three things can happen:

1. You get a set of answers to dwell on and contemplate and ask more whys about.
2. You don't get any answer or you get a wrong answer and this leads to a search for help to get to the bottom of it.
3. You create an excuse for why you are where you are, and you become a victim.

What are some things that all of these answers have in common? They keep you stuck. You still haven't done the thing that you wanted to do and now you are in the same place, only older. You have created other things to do that distract you from doing the

> *So what is the answer? Make your "shoulds" a must and do them. If you feel you can't, you must.*
>
> **– Tony Robbins**

thing that you wanted to do. See if you can follow this one: Instead of doing the task, you went to a place that is easier to deal with, the known past, and you avoided doing the thing you wanted to, the unknown. Many feel that it is easier to deal with the devil you know than the devil you don't.

Listen, you will meet with discomfort in this process. It's uncomfortable to stay in the same place for too long. It's also uncomfortable looking into the past for the crappy stuff that held you back. And it is uncomfortable to move forward and take on the unknown. So, you might as well take on the unknown and at least you'll be uncomfortable moving in the direction you want to go. Take bold steps in the direction you want to go and see where it leads you. Start with signing the following commitment. Thank you!

The Commitment

Here's the commitment. Please read and sign it. Once you do this, go online to www.dearoprahthebook.com and click on "my personal commitment." Enter your name and email and click on "I am committed." Your name will be added to the "I'm committed to my vibrant health and energy" list and if you choose, you will receive emails to help you. Your email address will only be used by me and can be removed any time.

I am committed to vibrant health and energy.

I will make choices that support this decision and adopt a lifestyle that will bring me the results I desire.

It is my right to live life fully and I now make choices that allow me to do so.

I will follow this guide and do what it takes.

Even when it's hard, I will do the right thing.

I believe in me.

_____   _____
Signature   *Date*

Congratulations! I am proud of you.

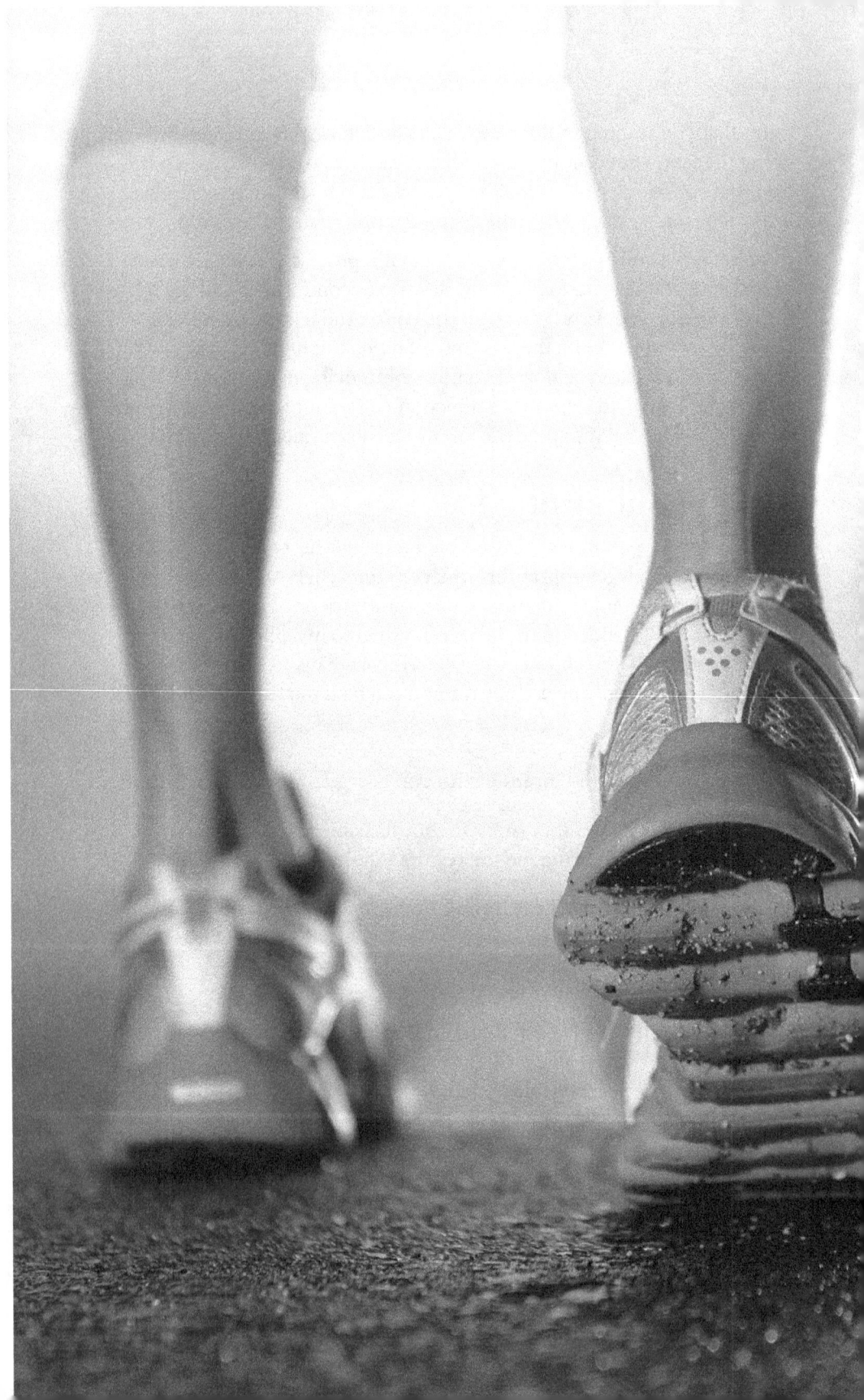

Section Two

Moving Towards Optimum Health

INTRODUCTION TO SECTION TWO:

In this section I'm going to talk about what to take into the body, toxins to avoid, exercise, positive attitude, and restoring your central nerve system—all of which can be made easy to do.

Remember, two keys to moving towards optimum health are: reducing your stress load and increasing your capacity to handle stress.

Reducing Stress Load and Increasing Your Capacity to Handle Stress

In the next chapters we will address the four parts that lead to a healthy lifestyle.

1. **The Way You Eat and What You Take into the Body:** nourishment – what you take into the body – food, supplements, water and air

2. **The Way You Move:** exercise

3. **The Way You Think:** positive mental attitude

4. **The Way You Take Care of Your Nerve System:** including chiropractic care

So, let's go and address what you should take into the body; including food, supplements and water!

CHAPTER SIX
What To Take into the Body:
Food, Water, Supplements

L et's take a look and see what you need to take into the body and what you need to leave out of the body in order to move you toward greater health and healing. Let's start with a key question.

Be thankful for what you have, you'll end up having more. If you concentrate on what you don't have, you never, ever have enough.

– Oprah

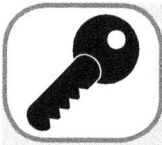

KEY QUESTION - What do you need to eat, drink and breathe in order to give your genes the best chance to produce and promote health and healing?

- Eat what the hunter-gathers ate and avoid processed foods
- Breathe the kind of air hunter-gathers breathed, when possible
- Drink non-polluted water

What To Take Into The Body: Food

Let's review genes. They haven't changed much in 20,000 years! If we roll time back that many years to examine what we were eating, drinking and breathing, we find we were eating:

- Nuts
- Berries
- Organic fruits and vegetables
- Free-range and organic meats
- Fish

We were breathing fresh air, unpolluted by "industry" and drinking fresh stream and river water that was moving and most likely replenished by rain. We didn't have to go to a shopping center to find a special section that contained these things. It was all that was there at the time. They had to put some effort out to get these foods and we still need to now.

And if we eat this way, our body will naturally express itself in health. And if you look at our hunter/gatherer ancestors or hunter/gatherers of today, for the most part, they don't have heart disease or diabetes. They have a little bit of cancer on occasion, and that's it.

You should get as much clean air as possible, drink as much clean water as you can find and eat organic fruits, vegetables and free-range meats or wild-caught fish from clean water sources.

If you look at what we're eating today, obviously, you'll see there's a big difference. And, you know, if it's not food, we shouldn't eat it! That's logical, right? In other words, if it's processed food, if it's in a box, it's probably not good for us because of all the added chemicals and preservatives.

How to Determine if Your Fruits and Vegetables Are Organic

Now that we have talked about what foods to avoid, let's talk about how to get those organic foods that are so much more nutritious than non-organic foods in vitamins and minerals (while avoiding the toxins). When you gather your fruits and vegetables in the grocery store, how do you know what's organic, what's genetically modified and what's industrially grown?

This is how you do it. First, find the tag or sticker. Usually there is an oval sticker on all of the fruits and vegetables. Second, notice that there is a number on the sticker. This is a code. This code is key to determining whether your produce is organic, genetically modified or commercially grown.

THE CODE

Commercially Grown	A four-number code
Example: ####	
Organic Grown	A five-number code that starts with 9
Example: 9####	
Genetically Modified	A five-number code that starts with 8
Example: 8####	(Unfortunately, not mandated to use at this time.)

A good way to remember this is to hate the 8 and love the 9.
Check it out next time you are in the grocery store.

GRAINS: Did your hunter/gatherers eat them?

Did they eat bread? No, they didn't. Grains were introduced in the agricultural age about ten thousand years ago. When we started to grow grains, we discovered we could make bread out of them and we also grew rice, wheat and other grains and ate those.

Are grains bad for you?

In my view, grains are not part of an ideal diet, but they are fine in moderation. You might argue that there's a huge community of Asians who have eaten rice for at least ten thousand years and they're some of the healthiest people on the planet. In the west, if the grains are of a high quality and you eat them sparingly, they'll be fine unless you have an allergy to one or more of them.

Are you allergic to some grains?

Wheat and corn have been added to so many of our foods that they have caused huge allergies, some with severe symptoms. One has to get grains in their purest form and avoid eating foods like commercial soups, where wheat gluten or wheat are often added. There are many processed foods that contain wheat and corn products. Do yourself a favor and avoid these. You might feel much better very soon.

What To Take Into The Body: Water

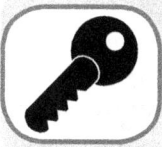

KEY QUESTION - What Kind of Water Is Best?

* Get the cleanest source of water possible.
* Avoid plastic containers for your water. Most plastic bottles leech bad chemicals into the water which create free radicals and can accelerate puberty and put hormones out of balance.
* Drink filtered water. Our water supply is full of junk these days.
* Add electrolytes to the water, especially when the temperature outside is hot—Himalayan Crystal Salt® can be added as it gives 84 minerals in almost identical ratios as exist in our bodies.

On a normal day, take the number of pounds you weigh, and divide it by 3. That is how many ounces of water you should drink in a day. So if you're 200 pounds, you would want to drink one third of that or about 66 ounces of water.

On a hot day or when you're exercising a lot, you would actually take the number of pounds you weigh and divide it by 2. Now if you are 200 pounds, you would want to drink one half of that or 100 ounces of water.

If you want to know how many glasses per day you need to drink that day, divide the number of ounces by 8.

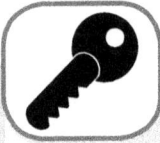

KEY QUESTION - How Much Water Do You Need To Drink?

Body Weight in lbs.	Ounces of water on a hot day (1/2 your body weight number)	Ounces of water on cool/inactive day (1/3 body weight number)
100 lbs.	50 ounces	33 ounces
120 lbs.	60 ounces	40 ounces
140 lbs.	70 ounces	46 ounces
150 lbs.	75 ounces	50 ounces
160 lbs.	80 ounces	55 ounces
170 lbs.	85 ounces	57 ounces

What To Take Into The Body: Supplements

Omega 3 Fatty Acids

Omega 3, 6 and 9 are all essential fatty acids which means we have to get it from our diet and we cannot make them ourselves. They are vital for normal metabolism.

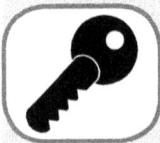

KEY QUESTION - What Supplements Do You Really Need To Take?

There are four major supplements that are vital for our bodies in this society at this time.

- Omega 3 fatty acids, preferably from fish oil
- A really good multiple vitamin
- Probiotics (acidophilus, bifidus and other good bacteria that need to be replenished in the gut)
- Vitamin D

Let's begin with the research on omega 3. Most of our meat is from animals that are grain and/or corn fed. There are three reasons why. First, it was found that farmers can get their livestock to market in about a year as opposed to the three years that it takes to get an animal fed on grass. So, by fattening them up quickly and getting them to market sooner, they make more money. However, the challenge is that cows aren't really designed to eat grain. And, like us, they weren't eating grain way back when. They were eating grass. Second, grain and corn is subsidized by the government, so it's cheap. Finally, free range farming may create healthier animals, but it takes up a lot more space than "modern" farmers can afford. How else can you get a 99 cent burger from a fast food place?

With grain-fed animals we get a much higher ratio of omega 6 fatty acids to omega 3. Now we need both omega 6 and 3 on a regular basis to form our cell membranes, to aid our hormonal and nerve systems among many other things. But they're supposed to be balanced at one to one, omega 6 to omega 3.

Many studies today have shown that our bodies can be out of balance as many as 30 to 1—omega 6 to omega 3, meaning there's 30 times the amount of omega 6 in our systems than there is omega 3. And this wreaks havoc on our systems and really throws us into a state of inflammation that can cause all kinds of problems. So what we need to do is supplement our diet with an omega 3 fatty acid. The main source in nature that we have of omega 3 fatty acids is fish. Unfortunately, our oceans and our streams are so polluted with mercury that it's very difficult to get the natural amount of omega 3 that we need because of the mercury that's built up in the fish.

There is hope, however. The best sources of omega 3 are derived from the small fish that are further down the food chain and that are freer of mercury. They catch them in Norway, for example, press them, distill them so that there's very little mercury and then bottle them. And that's how we get the best of our omega 3 supplement.

Not all omega 3 supplements are alike. We need to be very careful because there are a lot of them on the market. The first thing to avoid is altered or concentrated omega 3 fatty acids. Why should we alter nature? When have we ever done really well with changing nature when it comes to health?

If you do have an omega 3 supplement that you like, here is a test you should perform on it. If it comes in a gel form, poke a hole in it and smell it. If it smells rancid, throw it out, it's no good and will create free radicals. If you put it into a Styrofoam cup and it melts the cup, guess what, it is definitely not good for you!

There are many proponents of flax oil as a source of omega 3, 6 and even 9. But there is a problem around the metabolizing of flax seed oil. It needs a chemical to convert it to omega 3 fatty acids. And this chemical is in our body, but it depletes very rapidly when we start to take flax seed. So, there's not enough of that chemical to convert the flax seed into the omega 3 in the amounts we need to get the full benefits. Now flax seed is really good and we should take it, but as an exclusive supplement for omega 3, it's not going to do it. Fish oil, then, is the best source of omega 3. For omega 3 fish oil, I personally suggest Carlson's or Innate Choice brands at this writing.

Another way that you can help with your omega 3, omega 6 ratios is to buy free-range meats as much as possible. Here's the question you need to ask regarding free-range meats. Was it finished with grains or corn? Often times farmers will raise free range cattle and then fatten them up the last few weeks with grains and/or corn. This unfortunately alters the essential fatty acids ratios significantly.

Multi-Vitamin Supplements

It's clear that our food doesn't have nearly as many nutrients as it once did, even a hundred years ago, because the soil becomes depleted over time. Even with organic farming, it's very difficult to get all the nutrients necessary into our modern diet. So I highly recommend supplementing with a really good multi-vitamin. How do you choose a good multi-vitamin? As an interesting rule of thumb, a really good multi-vitamin is usually a really big pill and you have to take at least six of them a day. And they're fairly expensive.

However, that is not the only alternative, there is a much better one. Get food-based vitamins where possible. Ideally, get yourself a food-based product as opposed to a synthetic product. Avoid products that promise that you only need "one-a-day." Synthetic vitamins are not fully absorbable by the body and oftentimes can create imbalances because only part of the molecule you need is there. A beautiful piece of fruit, an orange for instance, has got Vitamin C, but it also has all the other things that help the Vitamin C work better in our bodies. And it comes as a complete package. A banana has potassium and everything else, but if you just take potassium, it can actually create imbalances as well, because it is lacking all the other things the banana has. So, for my bang for the buck, I go with something food-based. There are some really good food-based products out there. Standard Process makes an excellent food-based, multi-vitamin supplement. They absorb very well, they're balanced, and they give you the nutrients that you need in order to sustain health.

Another way for you to get the nutrients you need is to supplement your diet with juicing. Ideally you want to select a wide variety of organic fruits and vegetables for your juices. When you go into a supermarket or a farmer's market, select the brightest and most vibrant fruits and vegetables you can find. Consider your produce like a palette of paints, and use as many colors as you can.

Probiotics (or flora)

When we were hunter/gatherers, did we clean everything or did we pretty much eat it off the ground? Right, "off the ground!" That gave us enough natural bacteria (that existed in our environment) to coat and line our intestines. And that bacteria acted as a very good line of defense from invading bacteria and invading yeast.

That is what probiotics do for us, and we need to supplement it because our food is usually too clean. Flora, or probiotics, allow us to sustain our health. These good bacteria also produce some very important chemicals, like Vitamin K that we need in order to be healthy.

We have ten trillion cells in our body and we are supposed to have a hundred trillion bacteria in our body! Unfortunately, with all the antibiotics in our modern society and all the antibacterial products being used to clean hands and food, we deplete the good bacteria that we need in order to be healthy. So, it's very important to have a really good probiotic and there are wonderful brands out there. In fact, if you notice, probiotics are being put in our yogurt now. Don't use sugary yogurt or you'll feed the yeast in your body and sabotage the whole purpose of probiotics.

My two favorite brands of probiotics are Metagenics and Innate Choice.

Supplement with Vitamin D

Vitamin D is becoming very important because a lot of us tend to cover ourselves with sun screen when we go out in the sun. Sun is very important for our overall health, but when we cover ourselves with sunscreen, we don't allow the Vitamin D to be produced and that leads to all kinds of problems including osteoporosis.

A great source of vitamin D is cod liver oil. Once again, three great products are Carlson's, Innate Choice, and Biotics.

CHAPTER SEVEN
Toxins to Avoid: What You Don't Want to Take Into the Body

What *Not* To Take Into The Body: Toxins

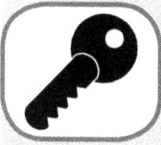

KEY QUESTION - What toxins do you need to avoid?

- Toxic foods
- Toxic food additives
- Toxic food preparations
- Toxins that go into the skin: touch-me-nots
- Toxins in personal hygiene products
- Household products
- Toxic environmental factors

TOXIC FOODS TO AVOID*

* All lists with asterisks in this chapter are courtesy of Dr. James L. Chestnut, B.Ed., M.Sc., D.C., C.C.W.P. (The Innate Diet™ & Natural Hygiene (pgs. 108-111))

[additional comments from me are italicized]

"The breakfast slimes, angel food cake, doughnuts and coffee, white bread and gravy cannot build an enduring nation."

– Martin H. Fischer, *German Physician*

1. Fried foods *(fries, donuts, chips that are fried, etc.)*

2. Processed & non-fiber carbohydrates *(flour, pasta, breads, etc.)*

3. Grains *[whole grains such as rice, whole oats, quinoa are okay in limited amounts]*

4. Dairy *[non-pasteurized dairy such as raw milk, raw kefir and raw butter are okay in limited amounts]*

5. Juices *[very diluted juices are okay in limited amounts]*

6. Caffeine *(in very limited amounts – I apologize to the addicts.)*

7. Sprayed, early harvest fruits and vegetables

8. Grain fed, antibiotic fed, hormone fed meats

9. Non-Filtered or non-distilled water *[unless derived from a clean stream]*

10. Dried fruits *(limited, organic only)*

11. Corn products

12. Soy products *(limited, if fermented – tempeh- miso)*

13. Shellfish *(bottom feeders – bioaccumulate toxins)*

14. Tuna [and other large fish] *(top of the food chain – bioaccumulate mercury)*

15. Farmed fish – higher toxicity – less omega 3, etc.

16. Smoked meats – full of nitrites and nitrates

17. Pork – high in parasites, mold spores in fat

18. Carnivores *(i.e. fish that eat other fish bioaccumulate [concentrate] toxins)*

19. Alcohol *(yes, even wine is bad)*

Eat, local, organic, non-processed food with plenty of vine-ripened local fruits and veggies, whenever possible.

Toxins To Avoid: Food Additives*

1. Hydrogenated fat

2. Partially-hydrogenated fat

3. Trans fats

4. Added salt

5. MSG

6. Hydrolyzed protein (disguised MSG)

7. Aspartame and other artificial sweeteners

8. Any and all chemical food additives and colors

9. Non-fiber carbohydrates (sugar)

10. Corn syrup or high fructose corn syrup

Toxins: Food Preparation Methods To Avoid*

1. Microwaves (banned in Russia!)
2. Non-stick pans
3. Frying with oils – add healthy oils after steaming or EAT it RAW
4. Fast cooking meats – better to slow cook
5. Boiling Vegetables – better to lightly steam or EAT them RAW

The Problem With Chemicals

The following is from an article titled PBS, Trade Secrets: The Problem (www.pbs.org/tradesecrets/problem/problem.html).

The chemical revolution from the last 50 years has altered nearly every aspect of our lives. Many of the products we rely upon every day – from plastic bags to computers – would not exist without synthetic chemicals. Most of us believe the chemicals in consumer products have been tested and approved by some government agency. In fact, until they are proven harmful, most chemicals are presumed safe.

Of the more than 75,000 chemicals registered with the Environmental Protection Agency, only a fraction have gone through complete testing to find out whether they might cause problems for human health. Many that are produced in enormous quantities have never been tested at all. Usually, it takes dramatic episodes of workplace injuries or wildlife poisonings, combined with rigorous scientific proof of harm and public outcry, before the government will act to restrict or ban any chemical. And that is no accident. The current regulatory system allows synthetic chemicals into our lives unless one is proven beyond doubt to be dangerous.

Today, while scientific research worldwide is finding that every one of us carries traces of synthetic chemicals in our bodies, scientists know very little about the risks of these low level exposures. We do know some chemicals are highly toxic. Some are carcinogenic. Others interfere with the reproductive system. Many others likely present no health threat at all.

The problem is that with most chemicals, we simply do not know how safe, or dangerous, they may be. They are everywhere around us – in the air, soil, and water; in our homes; and in our bodies. Not a single child today is born free of synthetic chemicals.

Toxins To Avoid: The Touch-Me-Nots Aka, "The Nasties!"

If you avoid these touch-me-not chemicals you will be so much better off, health wise. You may not have any idea what toll these chemicals take on your body. You've heard it before, your skin is the largest organ of your body. We take it for granted, but it really needs your awareness and a good routine of care.

The Nasties (Courtesy Of www.AbsolutelyPure.Com)

Avoid all of these in any products that touch your skin. Print and laminate this list to take with you shopping. Read the labels and do not buy products with the following in them.

- Isopropyl Alcohol
- Ethyl Alcohol, Methanol, Benzyl Alcohol, SD Alcohol and denatured Alcohol.
- Butyl, Ethyl, Methyl & Propyl Paraben
- DEA, MEA & TEA: (Diethanolamine, Monoethanolamine, Triethanolamine)
- Diazolidinyl Urea & Imidazolidinyl Urea
- FD&C Color Pigments

Synthetic Fragrances

- Mineral Oil, Liquid Paraffin (Paraffinum Liquidum)
- Petrolatum & Petroleum Jelly
- Polyethylene Glycol (PEG)
- Propylene Glycol (PG) & Butylene Glycol:
- Sodium Lauryl Sulfate (SLS) & Sodium Laureth Sulfate (SLES)
- Triclosan
- Phthalates

For a more detailed description of each of the above, see Appendix #2

Toxins To Avoid In Personal Hygiene

While we are talking about what is good and bad for your skin, let's discuss deodorant. Sweating is good and is one of the ways that your body gets rid of toxins. One of the main areas of discharge is your armpits. (By the way, remember that your skin is your biggest organ.) It has been speculated that one of the possible causes of breast cancer is the use of antiperspirants. Let's look at this.

You are meant to sweat. Most breast cancers occur at the root of the breast. This is located along the pectoralis minor muscle underneath your collar bone. If you block the sweat glands in the armpit, the toxins that would normally be excreted at the pit can back up. The place that it backs up to is the lymphatic system. There are many lymph nodes in the breast area along the root of the breast. Cancer is sometimes discovered in the lymph nodes when removed during lumpectomies and mastectomies.

So the theory here is that the toxic stuff that is supposed to be excreted at the arm pit gets backed up through the lymph system back into the breast tissue cells. I do not think that this has ever been officially proven, however the theory makes sense. So, doesn't it make sense to just not use an antiperspirant and use a deodorant that is organic and clean instead?

There are several good ones out there. Study "The Nasties" and avoid aluminum in your deodorants.

Another area of hygiene that must be discussed is bathing. When you wash with soap, you wash off the natural oils that are on your skin. Oils are good. Every day, your skin will replace those oils. Where do you think the oils come from? They come from inside your body. Unfortunately, this taking of oils from your body eventually leads to a deficiency in oils inside your body. Think about it. Did the Hunter-Gatherers bathe with soap?

The way to handle this: just wash the smelly parts daily with soap. If you like, you can still wash your entire body with soap once a week. By the way, as you begin to shift to a better diet, body odors lessen.

Toxins To Avoid: Household Toxins*

(courtesy of Dr. James L. Chestnut, B.Ed., MSc., D.C., The Innate Diet™ & Natural Hygiene)

1. Chemical cleaners
2. Chemical soaps and phosphate soaps
3. Dry cleaning chemicals
4. Chemical deodorizers
5. Anti-perspirants
6. Chemically perfumed deodorants
7. Chemical perfumes
8. Chemical hair products
9. Antibacterial soaps
10. Chlorinated bath and shower water – get a filter
11. Carpets
12. Chemical based paints
13. Vinyl siding and windows (PVC Poisoning)
14. Particle board and plywood (Glue is toxic and outgases for years
15. Fluoride in toothpaste and at the dentist

Toxins To Avoid: Environmental*

1. Closed car garages
2. Attached garages
3. Diesel fumes and gasoline fumes
4. Cigarette smoke
5. Lawn and garden pesticides and herbicides
6. Plastic food containers
7. Tracking industrial chemicals into house – take off your shoes!
8. Poor house ventilation – open windows and get air filters
9. Mercury in fillings, root canals, vaccines (flu especially)
10. Prescription and over the counter drugs
11. New cars (interior plastics outgas)
12. Fire retardants (in mattresses and baby clothes – highly toxic)
13. Cordless and cell phones

CHAPTER EIGHT
Exercise and Movement

Moving Toward Health and Healing

Everyday brings a chance for you to draw in a breath, kick off your shoes and dance.

– Oprah

KEY QUESTION - How Much Exercise Do You Need Per Day?

- Enough to counteract all the sitting you do
- Enough that is both safe for your age and condition
- Enough so that you feel considerably better mentally and physically
- Enough to challenge you

Exercise and Movement

If you were to look at hunter/gatherers to gauge how much exercise you need to really help your genes produce optimum health, what would you see? The hunter/gatherers moved around their environment about eight miles a day, on average. How long would it take you to walk eight miles a day, do you think? There's been lots of research saying all you really need is a half an hour of walking around a day. I don't agree.

One of the common questions that I ask in my practice is how many years have you been sitting more than three hours a day? Ask yourself that now. How many years have you been sitting more than three hours a day?

What would happen to a hunter/gatherer if they were sitting around three hours a day? They might become part of the food chain and not make it. We need to move around more. Being bold, I recommend 10 to 15 minutes of exercise for every hour of sitting you do depending on your fitness level. So, if you sit five hours at a computer, you need to exercise at least 50 minutes and preferably 1 hour and 15 minutes a day. If you sit eight hours, you need 1 hour 20 minutes to 2 hours of exercise a day. Now, you will get some of that shopping, or walking from place to place, but really, most people need more exercise than they get doing their normal activities.

What will motivate you to get more exercise? I have a suggestion: get a heart monitor or a pedometer and see how many miles a day you're actually moving around. Nike makes a wristband that not only keeps track of your distance but also can be plugged into your computer to track your progress. Or you can get a friend or family member to team up with in order to go walking on a regular basis. Or decide to run a marathon and get with a group to start to work yourself up to being able to run a marathon. There's lots of them around. Just go online and type in "training for the Boston (or LA etc.) marathon." And find a local group that will train you on a daily basis. You will gradually work up to running a marathon. It's amazing what you can do with the right commitment and training.

Challenge yourself. It will take effort and discipline, but the rewards are well worth it.

You may not have the time or opportunity to walk several miles a day. So I have a short cut for you. Find access to a machine—called The TurboSonic. This is a full body vibrational therapy machine developed by the Russian space program. The Russians found that the longer their cosmonauts were in space, the more bone density and muscle mass they lost. By standing on a vibrating plate for a certain duration per day, the cosmonauts were able to maintain their bone density and muscle mass while in zero gravity for a longer duration.

What this means for you is that you can have the benefits of a full workout by standing on a vibrational plate for about ten minutes a day. For more information about this kind of exercise see Appendix #4: Vibrational Therapy.

Adding Oxygen to Your Workout

What do you notice when athletes come to the sideline after a big play? Usually, they go right to the oxygen and inhale it. The reason is, oxygen allows athletes to recover faster

Benefits of TurboSonic Vibrational Exercise

- Gives you over an hour of cardiovascular workout in about ten minutes on the machine
- Can decrease the effects of stress
- Increases bone density
- Increases human growth hormone, dopamine and serotonin secretion
- Lowers cortisol and epinephrine secretion
- Enhances circulation
- Can reduce facial wrinkles
- As the frequency changes on this machine, it will actually work out different areas of your body.

so that they can get back to playing the game. When it comes to oxygen and exercise therapy, not only does oxygen allow you to recover faster, but it does a lot of other things as the list below will show. For those of you who want to lose weight, with more oxygen in your system, your body is able to burn calories faster and work more efficiently. Oxygen has an anti-aging effect as well.

The basic principles of exercise with oxygen therapy were discovered and studied by German physicians in the 1950s. They had their subjects breathe oxygen-enriched air of above 90% oxygen while exercising. And they found dramatic health benefits because it allowed the red blood cells and plasma to work at full capacity. So the German researchers showed that exercise with oxygen therapy is effective for various indications:

- for renormalizing the oxygen-loading of the blood
- for bettering lung function degenerated by old age and severe stress.
- for early stages of cataract
- glaucoma
- loss of field of vision
- impaired focus
- angina pectoris
- arrhythmias
- prophylaxis (preventative measures) and rehabilitation for heart disease
- edema
- peripheral circulation disorders (especially in the lower extremities)
- circulation disorders
- dizziness
- senile diabetes
- hypertension
- general acceleration of any rehabilitation program
- lasting increase in physical performance capacity
- defense stimulation
- immune system stimulation—especially after classical cancer treatments that use radiation or chemotherapy.

(For more information go to the official Exercise with Oxygen Therapy website: www.ewot.com)

When it comes to degenerative problems, such as anything from degenerative disc disease to cancer, lack of oxygen is a factor in all these conditions. If you can get more oxygen in the system, you can usually slow or even possibly stop or reverse these situations from happening. So, when it comes to degenerative conditions, the earlier you get oxygen into the system, the more positive the results. But if degeneration is too severe, there is a point of no return. In any case, you should always check with your doctor before getting oxygen therapy.

The Right Kind of Exercise

The right kind of exercise is key. It is important to learn good posture from professionally trained experts in the subject of posture and alignment. Some chiropractors, some highly trained personal trainers, and some Pilates and yoga instructors have gained this training. Research the training background of your instructors and make sure they pay very close attention to your proper alignment when you are exercising.

Dancers, for example, put a great deal of stress on their bodies doing certain leaps and other complex movements. If they have been trained correctly they can handle it, but if not, they can become injured.

Movement and Mental Attitude

Moving is not only about planned exercise, it includes how you move your body in all ways throughout the day. Moving is how you greet the world. It is how you move your ideas into the world and how you receive from the environment those things that "move" you to a better place.

Do you ever take the time to dance to some music, either privately or publicly? How do you pick up your children or embrace your friends or spouse? How do you walk down the street or into work? How do you approach and greet your clients, friends and family? Do you move with confidence, with a generous spirit, with the joy of living lifting your body up from the ground, rather than sinking into it heavily with every step?

The whole subject of exercise embraces the subject of posture. My editor, Susan Stroh, co-wrote a good book with Dr. Mike Spearman on this subject titled, *Change Your Posture, Change Your Life.* It is a vital subject to learn.

There is a higher truth about movement that is superior to just body mechanics and it includes how your movement expresses your truest, best self. Do you shuffle through life, eyes downward, or do you stride with confidence, head held high, eyes alert and looking outward, interested in your environment and the people in it? Just for fun, try this second alternative for an entire day and see what happens to your sense of well being and health.

In today's society people are spending much of their days texting, using their smart phones and, of course, doing massive time on the computer. These activities can put undue stress on bodies. The sedentary life has created all kinds of body problems that correct movement can solve.

As a parting thought for this chapter; you've heard people say, "That was a moving experience." Well, pun intended, your life should be a moving experience in all senses of the word!

CHAPTER NINE
Positive Thinking and Attitudes Lead to Greater Health and Healing

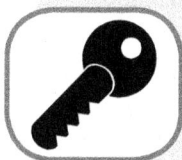

KEY QUESTION - How Do You Develop and Maintain a Positive Attitude?

I finally realized that to be grateful to my body was key to giving more love to myself.
– Oprah

- Engage in work that you like and be competent
- Stop listening to gossip, fear and generalities
- Stop watching/reading about bad news
- Fill up your cup everyday to overflowing
- Serve from your saucer not your cup
- Choose your friends and associates carefully
- Practice self-love and appreciation
- Practice love and appreciation of others
- Be playful. You might try giving yourself fun names that inspire you

Positive Mental Attitude—a closer look

How can you develop and maintain a positive attitude? I have listed some categories we will now consider.

Engage in work you love and be good at it

You spend a great part of your day working. It is important to love your work and be competent. This gives you satisfaction, high self-esteem and generates good feelings from your work associates and employers (or your patients and clients if you are self employed.) It is probably the number one way to develop a positive attitude. If you don't like your work, you really need to change that situation if at all possible. Do whatever it takes, whether you need to take courses to learn a new job until you can switch over or just choose another business with better working conditions and personnel. It is vital to your mental health and attitude.

Stop listening to gossip, fear and generalities

I'd like to remind you of a negative mental attitude in our society that is extremely unhealthy. I'm going to make a comparison between an attitude in nature and one in human nature.

Remember our zebra on the African plains that is getting chased by a lion? If you were there, you would have seen it running, running, running and suddenly out-running the lion and getting away. The lion stopped and went after some other animal. Remember what the zebra thought? She might have thought, *Whew, that was close.* And then maybe she thought, *Hey, there's some grass over there.* And she walks over and starts eating. The zebra gets over the event right away—end of chase, beginning of nourishment and relaxation.

What would someone in our society do if he or she were a zebra chased by a lion but managed to get away. Their friends and associates would hear about it for weeks, months, maybe years! It would be like,

"Oh, my gosh, did you see that lion? Oh, my goodness. It almost got me. Oh, gosh, it was terrifying."

And in hearing about it, people might race to their friends and say, "Wow, lions are all around, it's terrifying. They're all over and out to get us. Have you been chased by a lion, too? Oh, gosh, they're everywhere, they're everywhere. Oh, my gosh, Aunt Mabel was killed by a lion, too. They kill so many of us. It's horrific."

And then, that night it is all over the news: "Lions are coming into this area, they are EVERYWHERE! Lions are out to get us and are around every corner."

What does all this bad news, all the time, do for our health? It puts us into a constant state of stress. The news, in a majority of the cases, is negative and fear based. For instance, "Crime is on the rise, criminals are everywhere—out to get us. Criminals are here, criminals are there."

Stop watching/reading about bad news

This is a very harmful habit that must be consciously, vigorously stopped. How many of us, when we first get out of bed in that special part of the day when we are still half asleep and disarmed but our sub-conscious minds are on full alert, open the newspaper or turn on the news? This habit is harmful to our minds and bodies and opens us up to the grim, all-day-long habit of letting ourselves fill up with stress.

Then, after we have just been bludgeoned by the news that small businesses all over the country are folding, that the economy is not only bad but getting worse every minute, we go into our offices and see a pile of bills. And after we leaf through the pile of bills (which suddenly feels heavy and overwhelming) we wonder how long we'll be able to pay them until the bad economy devours our business, ourselves and our families.

Oh, but wait, there's more—then, we listen to our clients' bad news and our family members call us with bad news and our "friends" burden us with their problems and we listen to various other kinds of bad news all day long and then wonder why we are in a constant state of stress.

Fill your cup every day up to overflowing

It is vital to find ways to fill your cup every day. Fill it to overflowing. You can do it with affirmations, you can do it with prayer, with walking somewhere beautiful first thing in the morning, or by focusing your energy. There are so many different ways to overflow your cup that would be very helpful to you. I personally like setting and reviewing my goals and doing my affirmations first thing in the morning.

Another thing I find helpful and life affirming is to make sure I show my appreciation to the people on my team, my clients, my family and my resources. This can be done in a lot of creative ways—anything from an old fashioned thank you note to a public announcement on Facebook, to a little gift or bonus.

These are all key, powerful things that can overflow you and turn on your light for the day so that you're going out there attracting all the good things in life. So that's what positive mental attitude is all about—making sure that you're full to overflowing and refusing to fill yourself with bad news. When you are full to overflowing, you have no space for bad news anyway. You are too busy serving, being a source of good news, of healing, of good information, of life-affirming energy.

Serve from your saucer and not from your cup

One of my favorite sayings is, "Always serve from the saucer and not from the cup." (Lisa Nichols) This is really what we're talking about when we talk about positive mental attitude. Let's define your cup as what holds your positive energy allotment for the day. You start the day off with your cup half full and you begin serving throughout the day. About two or three o'clock your cup is empty and you get grumpy and life becomes less fun for you and everyone around you!

Let's start your day in another way. You fill yourself up in the morning to overflowing by goal setting, positive affirmations, visualization, listening to great music, dancing naked in front of the mirror, reading something inspiring and so on. The overflow fills your saucer. Now, throughout the day, you serve from your saucer and at the end of the day, your cup is still full and you feel good and so do people around you.

Choose your friends and associates carefully

Someone once said that you are most like the five people you hang around with most of the time. So, if you find that you're around a bunch of negative people, you may want to start shifting and changing who you spend time with. If you can, bring your friends with you, lift them up. But if you can't, you may have to leave them behind. You want to be around positive people who are focused, optimistic, doing well and who support your dreams. You'll live longer if you have a positive mental attitude and surround yourself with people who have the same.

Develop an attitude of self love and appreciation

Your love and appreciation for others must start with appreciation of yourself. We are here, in my opinion, to express our love in ways that we discover fit our purposes, interests, values and abilities.

Develop an attitude of love and appreciation toward others

A positive mental attitude comes down to love and appreciation. When you don't recognize love in your life, you get stress. Appreciation lifts you out of negative situations. If, for example, you are having a dispute with your neighbor, find out what is right and good about them, put your attention on these things and your animosity will dissipate.

Be playful. A fun way to inspire a positive attitude—playful self-naming

I knew a woman who once called herself "Vibrant Vixen" because she wanted vibrant energy and power. When a situation came up, she would ask herself, "What would Vibrant Vixen do in this case?" For example, when she was ordering food, as the Vibrant Vixen, she'd make choices off the menu that would enhance her power so she could have more vibrancy. Or, if she were considering whether or not to exercise, she would ask herself,

"What would the Vibrant Vixen do?" Then she would choose to go exercise.

What playful name, that will inspire a positive attitude, might you choose for yourself? Are you the "Scintillating Storyteller"? "Competent Charlie" or "Cheerful Cheryl"? Are you "Animated Adam"? "Inspiring Iris"? "Great Ideas Granny"? "Lean Leonard"? "Brilliant Barbara"? "Talented Tomas"? "Shimmering Sandy"? Are you "Calming Carl," who lifts people out of the doldrums with his help? Are you "Trouble-Shooter Terry"? "Hope-Giving Hank"? "Humorous Hal" What name would help you grow into that vision you have of your ideal self?

Besides choosing a name for yourself, you could pick a theme for a day, a week, a month or a year. For example, I chose a theme for this month: "Practice Authentic Self-Expression." Whenever I get the chance, I express my individuality expansively and watch how that benefits people around me.

Here's a quote from Oprah that I love!

> ## What we're all striving for is authenticity, a spirit-to-spirit connection.– *Oprah*

CHAPTER TEN
Get More Out of Life—
Restore Your Nerve System

Many of you have already been to a chiropractor. Some of you, maybe even more than one chiropractor. But have you ever been to a "neurologically-based wellness chiropractor?" What I mean by that is someone who is not only interested

My philosophy is that not only are you responsible for your life, but doing the best at this moment puts you in the best place for the next moment.
– Oprah

in your nerve system but also how your lifestyle affects your nerve system as well. This book is really about improving your lifestyle with the purpose of enhancing your nerve system. By the end of this chapter will understand why your nerve system is so important to keep you healthy and well for a lifetime and how chiropractic care can help you with that.

The Benefits of Chiropractic Care

Chiropractic care increases your capacity to handle stress and helps you restore your nerve system to optimum function.

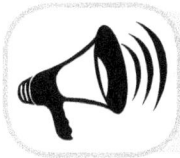

Chiropractic Care Does Two Things:
- It increases your ability to handle stress
- It reduces your stress load

How Does Chiropractic Care Increase Your Capacity To Handle Stress?

In previous chapters we discussed how you can reduce your stress load by what you eat, drink, put on your skin, through avoiding environmental toxins and finally through the proper exercise. Another way to reduce your stress is through chiropractic care. Mainly, it does so by relieving pressure and stress that is impinging on the nerve system and by getting the body into a more proper alignment so that it can let go of stresses more easily and operate more efficiently.

Chiropractic care enables your body to use less energy to do the same functions as before you had the adjustment.

An interesting research study was done where they gave a patient a functional MRI that measures brain activity. (*Journal of Vertebral Subluxation Research*, 1998; 2(1): Cover) They said, "Move your foot." So the subject moved her foot and they measured how much brain activity it took to move her foot. They took her out and gave her a specific chiropractic adjustment. Then they put her back into the functional MRI and said, "Move your foot." It actually took 1/20th the brain activity to move her foot after the adjustment. In other words, she became that much more efficient in her nerve system.

To express this another way, imagine yourself driving in Southern California on the 405 freeway during rush hour. The 405 is one of the most highly congested roadways in the world. The traffic is rush-hour hell all the time! Let's say you're stuck on the 405, going 0 to 2 miles per hour and it's extremely stressful. What if, all of a sudden, I came along and snapped my fingers and 95% of all of the cars were gone—just all cleared out. What would that do to your drive? Are you less stressed? Of course, you'd be less stressed. You'll be able to get where you want to go more efficiently, more easily and more quickly. That's what chiropractic care is about. That's the "1/20th of the effort" effect. Based on this research, a chiropractic adjustment can eliminate 95% of the static that's built up in your nerve system due to subluxation (interference in the nerve system usually caused by misalignment of spinal bones.) Can you see how this could increase your capacity to handle stress?

Using the analogy of hardware and software systems related to the spine and central nerve system, let's further see how chiropractic care can help.

The hardware system consists of the structural support of the body: including bones, discs, fascial, ligaments and muscles—how they move and how they operate. The hardware system can exert considerable pressure on the nerves. The joints and discs need to keep moving. As they move they become nourished. If they don't move, they break down.

How does chiropractic care help reduce stress in your hardware system?

Through adjustment, pressure can be relieved in your hardware system. And your chiropractor can help you find the right exercise and nutrition programs to keep your joints and discs moving.

---

1   Fascia - A sheet or band of fibrous connective tissue enveloping, separating, or binding together muscles, organs, and other soft structures of the body. (The American Heritage® Dictionary of the English Language, Fourth Edition copyright©2000 by Houghton Mifflin Company. Updated in 2009. Published by Houghton Mifflin Company. All rights reserved.)

The software system consists of the programs that are running within the nerve system which provide the flow of information transferred from one point to another throughout the nerve system. So the software system allows your body to run without much conscious brain in-put. There are programs which enable messages that go from the brain to other parts of the body and back to the brain. Most of the software programs (continuing the analogy to computers) run in the background. They usually run on a reflex-type basis. These programs are working in the nerve system 24/7, keeping us alive and in balance.

In other words, your nerve system, consisting of your brain, spinal cord and nerves, controls and coordinates every single function in your body and brain. In fact, there are over 200,000 nerve impulses per second that travel from your brain, down your spinal cord, through the nerves, to and from every cell of your body. Without thinking about it at all, your hair grows, your heart beats, you digest your food, you breathe through your lungs, you experience all your emotions, and even think your thoughts, while your central nerve system controls and coordinates all these functions. You literally live your life through your nerve system. Every function in your body and all of your senses are completely dependent on your nerve system.

How does chiropractic care get rid of accumulated static in the software of your body?

What is Static? When I say "static," I mean the accumulation of all the aberrant, learned behaviors running in the background. When we become injured, the body goes out of balance and the longer the imbalance continues, the longer it becomes ingrained as a pattern in our nervous system. Similarly, if we eat the same junk food over and over again, we create an imbalance which causes cravings for more junk food. The resultant eating of junk food is reinforced and becomes what is known as a bad habit. These are ways things can get stuck in our nerve system.

You know when you get a brand new computer—how it runs like a charm, quickly flowing from program to program? Then after a few months or maybe even a year, you notice it's slowing down, not running as well. You discover some quirks and have to call tech support. What you usually find (or your computer technician finds) are random programs that have attached themselves to your computer and are running in the background. There might be a virus or two as well.

As these programs accumulate, layer upon layer in our computers, we will put up with it for a while or occasionally, for way too long, until a crash occurs or until we simply lose something we value. So we make the emergency call to our computer technician or tech support and, if we're lucky, the computer professional can clean up the viruses, the accumulated software and get rid of the spam and junk. If we are not so lucky, we may have lost an entire hard drive which results in great expense and time to recover the data in it. This time away from our computers is not only annoying but could eat into our incomes. We might even need a whole new computer.

When the "software" programs accumulate in the background in your body, you may experience a slowing down, a bogging down and even a breaking down. In chiropractic we call this "dis-ease."

When you know you're slowing down and the body is not running as smoothly as usual, seek chiropractic care immediately—your doctor of chiropractic can more readily restore your nerve system function if you get there early. However, if you wait until you breakdown, can't get out of bed because of severe pain, for example, your chiropractor will need more visits to restore your nerve system and to balance your body. This is added expense and time and sometimes impacts your ability to work, earn income and enjoy your life. Unlike your computer, you only have one body.

Most people have discovered the time, money and stress-saving benefits of having a computer maintenance program so that they never have to experience a slow down in their computer's efficiency. Likewise, more and more individuals are realizing the importance of chiropractic support designed to allow them to be proactive so they can experience peak efficiency, performance and mental clarity for optimum productivity and life expression.

Summary of harmful "software" running in the body

New programs get installed or else tweaked every time there is an injury or insult to the body.

If somebody breaks an ankle and they get it reset, for six weeks, they're walking in a cast. That new way of moving with a cast is now programmed into your nerve system, and that's what it becomes—the new way you will now move.

The body compensates for injuries or illnesses with learned patterns accumulated over the years. These may have helped us survive at the time but are now attached as solutions, programmed in, that actually slow us down and make our functions less efficient. In addition to these programs running in the background, if we add stress to this bogged-down system, we start to fall apart and we call this condition, dis-ease.

Defining "Subluxation"

Subluxation is an adaptive response within the nerve system to an overload of stress; be it chemical, physical or emotional. As this adaptation (or subluxation) continues for a long time, the spine and nerve system become damaged. Once damage is done to the bones and structures around the joints of the spine, intervention is required and may be necessary for a lifetime depending on the amount of damage done. Ideally, one should seek care long before damage occurs or when one becomes first aware that something is wrong. The proactive person recognizes that they live in a stressful environment, and chooses to seek chiropractic care for prevention purposes before experiencing any symptoms. However, in our society most people choose to seek care after the symptoms have become so bad, that it's an emergency.

Subluxation, then, is a nerve interference created by your innate intelligence (your master operating system or governing body) to allow your system to adapt to an overload of stress. Much like a dimmer switch, it will dim down the signal, thus allowing you to function without dire consequence while under your stress overload. This is meant to be short term. But as the stressors continue on and on, the dimmer switch dims more and more, and eventually symptoms will develop that are meant to tell you that something needs to change—now! These symptoms are usually in the form of back tension that leads to pain, neck pain, headaches, digestive problems, fogginess, asthma and reproductive issues (just to name a few) all depending on where the nerves go that are most affected.

The results of your chiropractic care will be in direct proportion to the quality of your lifestyle. In other words, if a person doesn't let go of bad habits, the chiropractic care will not be as effective. However, if you change your bad habits into good habits, your chiropractic care will be much more effective. Often, I've seen that once a person starts chiropractic care, lifestyle changes become more attractive and he/she finds the discipline to make the changes that will better their overall health.

Reducing Your Stress Load through Motion:
Why Movement Is So Important in Chiropractic Care

In our chapter on exercise and movement, we emphasized how very important it is for you to move a great deal. Bodies were not designed to be sedentary. In this chapter, I want to underscore how movement is vitally important to the care of your nerve system and how it relates to chiropractic and medical care.

Do you have a "back problem" or a "health problem"?

Subluxations (nerve interference or damage) cause body and mind miscommunication malfunction and dis-ease.

CHIROPRACTIC PREMISE

1) Your nervous system (brain, spinal cord and nerves) controls and coordinates everything in your body and mind.
2) When your nerve energy flows abundantly without obstruction, your body and mind are 100% self-communicating, self-healing, self-regulating and robust.
3) When subluxations (nerve interference or damage) impede nerve flow, similar to static on your cell phone, you are no longer functioning at 100% and your health and vitality are compromised.
4) Subluxations are caused by our inability to handle life's three major stressors; physical, mental-emotional and chemical.
5) Left uncorrected, subluxations have devastating effects upon human health and well-being, leading to breakdown, malfunction and dis-ease.
6) Our goal is to locate subluxations, remove them and their causes and allow you to heal yourself on every level.
7) Only chiropractors can determine if you have subluxations. WHO DO YOU KNOW THAT NEEDS TO BE CHECKED?

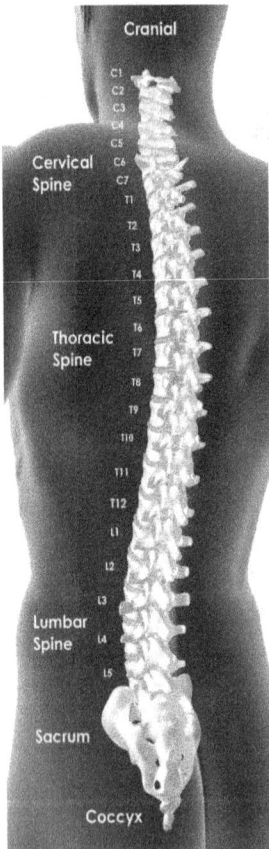

SPINAL LEVEL	BODY PAIN	INTERNAL ORGAN OR BODY FUNCTION	COMMON INTERNAL SYMPTOMS POTENTIALLY INDICATING MALFUNCTION or "DIS-EASE"
Cranial C1, 2	Headache	All anatomical structures within the head; Brain, Cranial Nerves, Eyes, Ears, Nose, Throat, Sinuses, etc.	Spacey, dizzy, low energy, memory trouble, brain fog, ADD, ADHD, ear aches, tinnitus, nose bleeds, sinus problems, snoring, sleep disorders, sore throats, colds, influenzas, itchy & achy eyes, allergies, food sensitivity
C3	Neck	Diaphragm	Difficult to take a deep breath, chronic fatigue, anxiety, vertigo, shortness of breath, allergies
C4		Thyroid	Low = weight gain, feelings of being cold High = insomnia, nervousness, swollen glands
C5	Shoulder	Sugar Handling Function	Craving sweets, tired after eating, headaches if too long between meals, emotional instability, heart palpitations
C6	Arm	Stomach	Stomach pains after eating, needs antacids
C7	Hand	Liver	Sluggishness, sneezing, nightmares, burning feet, allergies
T1, 2	Finger	Heart	Coronary artery disease, functional heart conditions, high or low blood pressure, chest pain
T3		Lungs & Bronchi	Asthma, shortness of breath, chronic coughs, allergies
T4	Upper back	Gall Bladder	Heartburn, bloating after meals, gassy, burping, trouble with fatty foods
T5		Stomach	Heartburn, indigestion, stomach troubles, ulcers
T6		Pancreas	Craving sweets, indigestion, tired after eating, heart palpitations, emotional instability, headaches if too long between meals,
T7	Mid back	Spleen & Immune Function	Lowered resistance, immune deficiencies, frequent colds or influenzas, allergies
T8		Liver	Headaches, low energy, sneezing, nightmares, burning feet
T9		Adrenal Glands	Overwhelmed by stress, allergies
T10		Small Intestine	Digestive complaints: 1-2 hours after eating
T11, 12		Kidneys & Bladder	Decreased urine output, swollen ankles, puffy eyelids, kidney or bladder infections, high or low blood pressure
L1	Low back	Ileocecal Valve	Bad breath, flatulence, headaches when sleeping too long, dark circles under the eyes, toxicity, allergies
L2	Hip	Cecum	Digestive complaints: 1-2 hours after eating, abdominal cramps, allergies
L3	Leg	Endocrine Glands: Thyroid Pancreas, Liver, Adrenals	See organs' primary subluxation sites: C4, C5, C7, T6, T8
L4, 5	Knee, Ankle	Colon, Prostate or Uterus	Bowel problems, coated tongue, headaches, allergies, hemorrhoids, varicose veins, prostate problems, impotence, dysmenorrhea, PMS, menopause symptoms
Sacrum	Foot	Reproductive Organs	Reproductive disorders
Coccyx	Toe	Overall tone of the nervous system	Chronic depression, migraines, vertigo, dyslexia, epilepsy, ADD, ADHD, compulsive disorders, sensitivity to light, PMS, dysmenorrhea, menopause symptoms, impotence

Spine figure labels: Cranial, Cervical Spine (C1–C7), Thoracic Spine (T1–T12), Lumbar Spine (L1–L5), Sacrum, Coccyx

Adjustments correct subluxations so your body can heal and function at higher levels.

REFERENCES: Fix, J. D., Ph.D, Neuroanatomy, 3rd Edition, Lippincott Williams & Wilkins, 2002; Kandel, E.R., Schwartz, J.H., Jessell, T.M., Principles of Neural Science, Appleton & Lange, 1991; Hoppenfeld, S. M.D., Physical Examination of the Spine and Extremities, Appleton-Century-Crofts, 1976. Netter, F.H. M.D., The CIBA Collection of Medical Illustrations, Vol 1, Nervous System, Part 1, Anatomy and Physiology, Ciba Pharmaceuticals Division, Ciba-Geigy Corp, 1991. * This chart has been simplified for demonstrative purposes. It does not illustrate all intricate nerve pathways. The symptoms listed are a guide to potential effects of subluxations. * Special thanks and recognition to Dr. Nicolai Lennox and Dr. Gurutrang Singh Khalsa in the creation of this chart. © Rosen Coaching, Inc. (800) 876-8384

Medical research has shown that when the motion of the joints is diminished (subluxation), after 14 days without correction, the joints show signs of degeneration. (*Experimental Osteoarthritis in the Rabbit*: by Tapio Videman published in *Acta orthop. scand.* 53, 339-347, 1982) Most medical doctors know this and so, to avoid degeneration after surgery, they now insist that their patients are up and walking around as soon as possible.

After the age of 13, we lose our blood supply to our discs. Therefore they are fed by motion. So in order for there to be nourishment to the discs there has to be movement for fluid to be able to move in and out of the discs. When you are subluxated, the joints get stuck and become unable to move properly.

How Movement Is Related to the Anatomy of Your Discs

The discs are the shock absorbers between your vertebrae, that allow you to move around and while doing so, they absorb some of the stress that occurs as you sit, bend, lift, walk, run and jump. As stated above, before age 13, your discs are fed by your blood supply, after age 13, they are hydrated and nourished through motion. Motion ensures the discs keep hydrated, energized and working correctly.

The Spine and Its Joints

Joints consist of two bones and the connective tissue between them. In the case of the vertebrae, they are separated by the disc as well as by two other joints forming a tripod of support.

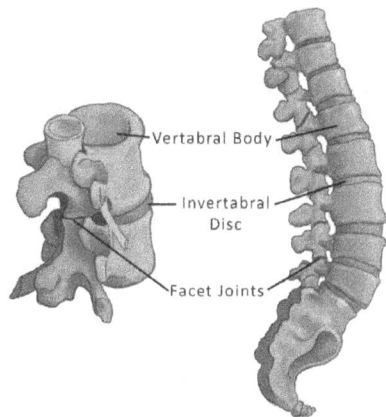

When a subluxation occurs, the body will lock the joints in that area as a protection, using the muscles around the joint to do this. Over time, scar tissue develops around the joints further locking them down. The lack of motion doesn't allow for nourishment to enter the discs and so eventually the whole joint and the nerves begin to deteriorate.

Repairing, Restoring and Preventing

The goal of chiropractic is to repair the damage of long standing subluxation, restore the function of the damaged nerves and teach you ways that you can stop recreating the problem.

To help you repair the damage or even prevent problems from happening, we will now teach you some passive exercises. When you actively exercise, you are consciously moving your body around. Unfortunately, when you do this, the subluxated joints still stay locked down. So, the way to get around the locked muscles and joints is to do passive exercises.

Exercise and Chiropractic Care—Why Passive Exercises are Important

Passive exercises are exercises that use one body part or parts to move another body part. For example, in an active twist of the spine, one might turn your body using the muscles of your spine to twist. A passive exercise to stretch your spine, if you are seated for example, is where you use one arm to push off the table as you turn your torso and pull on the chair back with the other arm to get your spine to twist and to hold that position. As you relax through your spine and use your arms to turn, that passive exercise allows movement in areas that aren't normally able to move because they're locked down due to subluxation.

By doing these passive exercises throughout each day, you actually make sure that you get more fluid and more hydration into your discs so that they can heal.

If you teach children to do this habitually when they are young, as they grow and continue to do passive exercises, their spinal health will most likely remain very good. Chiropractic care, in combination with these exercises, is key to rejuvenating the hardware of your spine.

For a sheet of the exercises that you can print up and put on your fridge, go to www.dearoprahthebook.com.

PASSIVE HOME EXERCISE PROGRAM FOR SPINAL HEALTH

General Rules:

1. Stretch only to a feeling of discomfort, not pain; if you experience pain, STOP.

2. Do not bounce.

3. Breathe throughout your stretches – do not hold your breath.

4. The idea is NOT to pop your back, but to stretch.

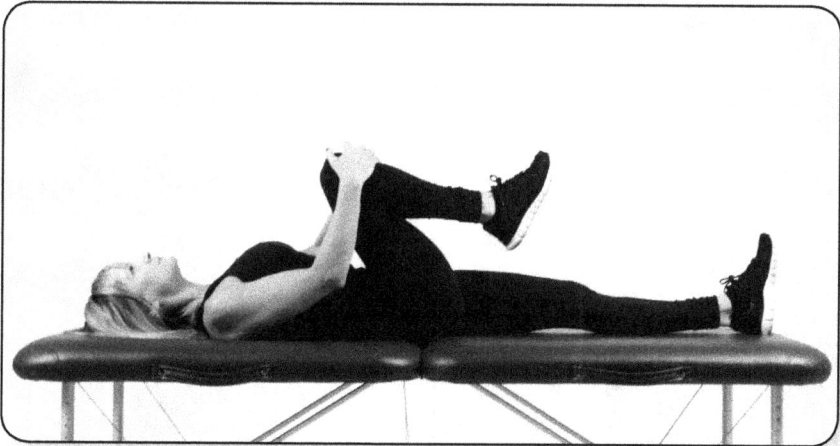

1. Knee-to-Chest Stretches

*   Lie on your back and bring your bent knee to your chest, holding it with your hands for 5 seconds.

*   Repeat on the other side.

*   Do this for a total of 3 times.

*   <u>Do this exercise 3 times per day.</u>

2. Seated Trunk Rotation Exercise

- Sit on the edge of a chair with your feet flat on the ground. (Or sit on the side of your bed with your feet flat on the floor.)

- Place your right hand on your left knee, and your left hand behind you. Use your arms to gently rotate your upper body towards the left, and turn your head to the left as well.

- Hold for 5 seconds.

- Repeat on right side.

- Do this for a total of 3 times.

- <u>Do this exercise 6 times per day.</u>

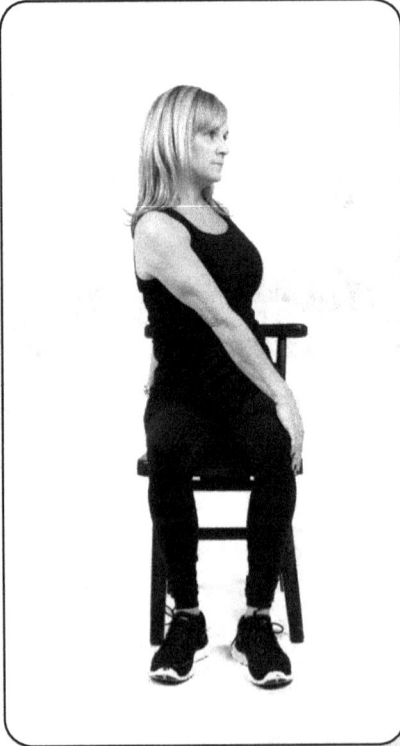
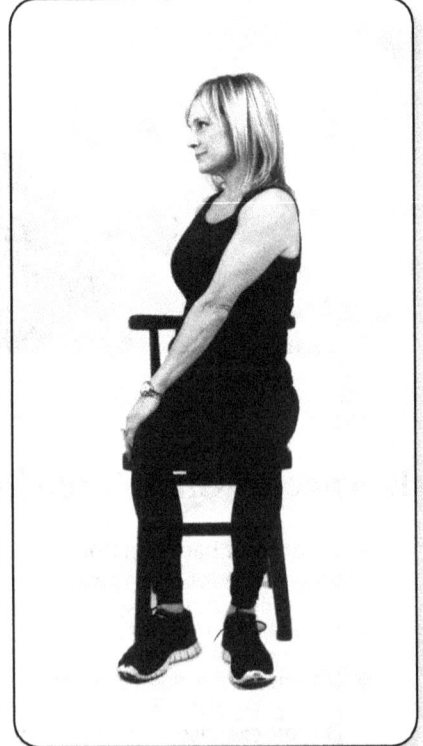

3. Neck Stretches

- While sitting upright, turn your head to the right.
- Using your left hand, apply gentle pressure to your left cheekbone, pushing your head into further right rotation.
- Hold this position for 5 seconds.
- Repeat on the left using the right hand on the right cheekbone.
- Do this for a total of 3 times.
- Repeat this exercise 6 times per day.

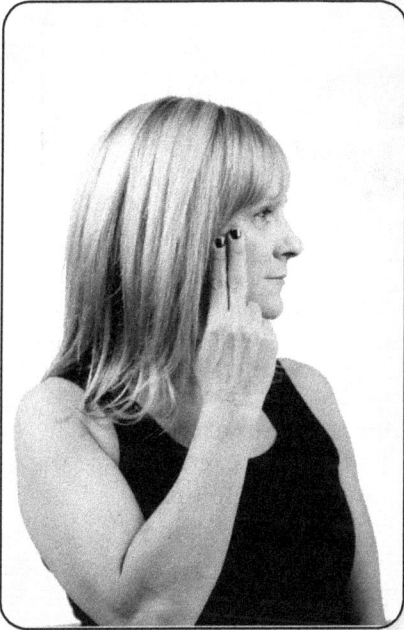

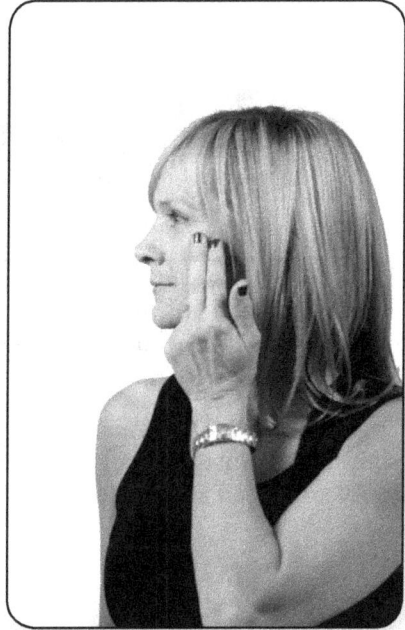

4. Standing Tall Exercise

- Lie on your back with your heels, buttocks and back of head resting against the floor.

- Lift both arms up so that your armpits form a 90-degree angle to your body.

- Lift your hands up so that the backs of your hands approximate the floor and your elbows form a 90-degree angle.

- Hold this for 60 seconds.

- Repeat this exercise 3 times per day.

Special note #1: You may need to work up to 60 seconds and you may even find you cannot put your hands back against the floor at first. Keep

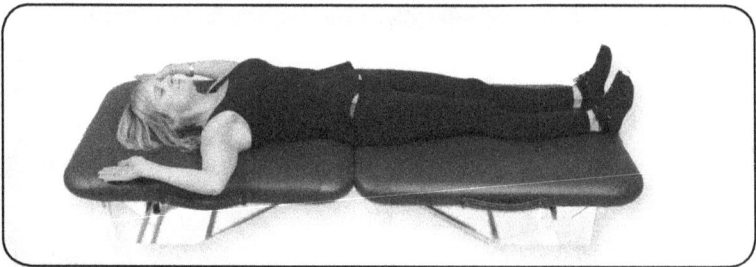

working at it and little by little you may be able to do it. This exercise is meant to combat the hunched back-forward head posture we see in most seniors.

Special note #2: Dr. James L. Chestnut teaches this exercise as standing against the wall instead of the floor. His exercise is for the more advanced student/patient. You can work up to this.

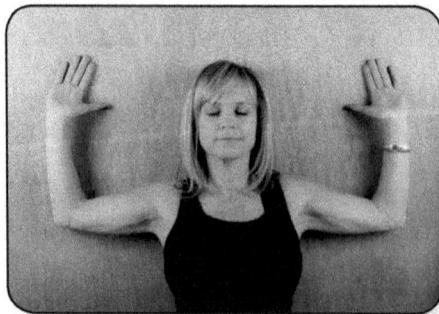

(Can Be Added after You
Master the Above)

5. Cat Stretch

- Get on the floor on your hands and knees with your hands under your shoulders, your knees under your hips.

- Arch your back upwards dropping your head between your arms, like a cat stretching.

- Gently rock from side to side adding passive motion throughout your back.

- Do this for a slow count of 10.

- Repeat twice a day.

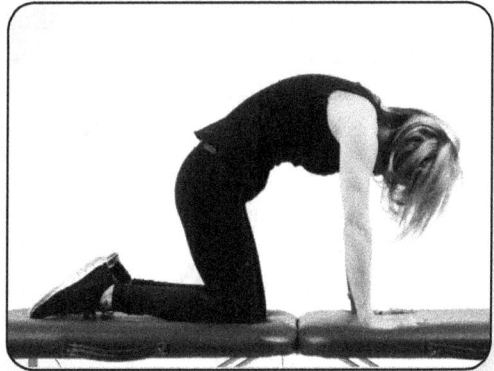

6. Knee-to-Shoulder Stretches

- Lie on your back and bring your knee up to your chest, towards the opposite shoulder. You should feel a stretch into your buttocks area.

- Hold for 5 seconds.

- Repeat on the other side.

- Do this a total of 3 times

- Repeat this exercise 2 times per day.

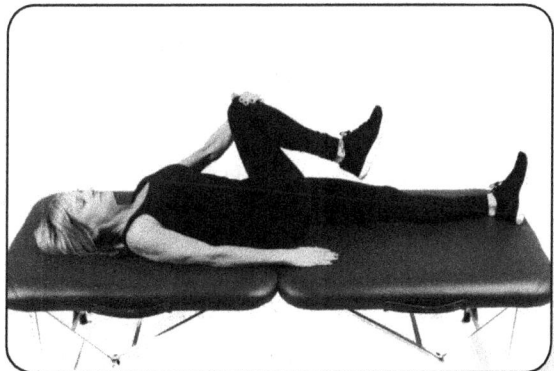

Summary of the Role of the Chiropractor

Chiropractic care is meant to repair the damage to the joints and nerves that has accumulated due to physical, chemical and/or emotional stress. The best chiropractors also teach you how to stop recreating subluxations by utilizing many of the lifestyle ideas, that you've learned in this book, designed to reduce your stress load. Your chiropractor may also advise you on what kind of specific nutritional supplementation you may need and how to do the right kind of exercises to regenerate your joints and discs and keep them healthy.

You have as a goal, health and healing. You achieve this by both reducing your stress load and increasing your ability to handle stress. In this culture at this time, it takes conscious effort, discipline and the right practitioners and friends to support your game of achieving optimal health for you and your body.

Not surprisingly, we have to work at getting and staying healthy in different ways than we did when we were hunter/gatherers. Before, we had to hunt and gather and just avoid the stuff that would kill us. In our modern civilizations, however, all our food is readily available, but we have to "hunt" for the healthy foods and learn how to avoid those foods and products that could kill us.

I contend that if you do the following, you will achieve great health.

- Avoid toxins in the environment.
- Give your body the right foods, water and supplements.
- Do the correct exercises for *your* body.
- Get and maintain chiropractic care to repair any damage or to prevent any potential damage to your nerve system.
- Create and maintain a positive mental and/or spiritual attitude.
- Choose your friends and associates carefully so as to surround yourself with people supportive of your new lifestyle and goals.

If you look at the most successful business people, artists, persons of any profession who also glow with health and contribute in a way that enhances those around them, you will find they have chosen an exceptional team of health practitioners. They will have the top chiropractors, nutritionists, exercise teachers or personal trainers, massage therapists, holistic dentists and doctors and very positive friends and associates.

You might say, "Yes, but they are wealthy." Not necessarily. I know a woman who exchanges her business expertise for massage, chiropractic and nutritional work. If it is important enough to you, you will find a way.

Just remember, though, even with an exceptional team of practitioners, you still have to do the work!

In the next chapter, you will learn how to get the most out of your relationship with your chiropractor.

CHAPTER ELEVEN
When to Go to a Chiropractor

The simple answer is, make an appointment now! People usually wait until it gets so bad they feel they have no choice but to do something about it. That's part of the programming of our society: somehow, we get the idea that we need to buck up and wait until it is so painful we have to seek help. You hear the saying, "If it's not broke don't fix it." This is not a good philosophy when it comes to bodies. Why?

The Surprising 10% Fact

Only 10% of the nerve system has to do with what you *feel*. And the other 90% has to do with function. So, if you wait until you actually *feel* pain, it's most likely been going on and altering your function for quite a while. You can not rely on your feelings when it comes to your nerve system or your health.

Take an example from dentistry. Let's say you go to the dentist and they find a cavity. Did you have that cavity yesterday? Of course, you did! Research shows that it can take up to 15 years for you to feel the cavity. In other words it could take that long for the cavity to touch a nerve so that you notice it.

Here's another example, the worst case scenario – pancreatic cancer. This particular cancer can hang out in the body for years until the person finally feels it, and then it's most likely too late to cure it.

Get your nerve system checked before you feel a problem.

How Often Do You Need to Go to a Chiropractor?

If you insist in believing that you only need to get chiropractic care when it really hurts, you'll eventually find a chiropractor who will tell you what you want to hear, "Come back when it hurts." But that's not what you *need* to hear. And I'm just telling you what the current research shows and it's very real. In fact, all chiropractors up on this research want to see their patients at least every two weeks—to avoid any further degeneration from life's stresses and strains.

In Southern California, where people are being bombarded by various stressors such as pollution, I recommend at least once-a-week checkups to keep ahead of the degeneration and to correct subluxations accumulated from the past. You want to increase your capacity to handle stress, right? Well, subluxations are a great source of stress, so without them you immediately have more strength and attention to live the life you want to live as well as to handle other stresses.

Do You Have to Continue Chiropractic Care for the Rest of Your Life?

The short answer is yes. Now, before you get discouraged about this, let me remind you about something you already know. You know you have to brush your teeth daily and floss the ones you want to keep, right? You know you have to eat the right foods and drink water every day to survive, correct? And you know you have to exercise daily. If you ever had orthodontia treatment, you know that after you got the braces off, you wore a retainer to prevent the teeth from moving back into the faulty way they were.

Here's another analogy: If a person is diagnosed with heart disease, when does he or she ever stop checking their blood pressure or getting their blood work redone? They never do. They go to the doctor regularly to make sure their hearts are working well. A similar thing is required for those with degenerative disc disease. This condition is a form of arthritis and results from subluxations that have been neglected for a long, long period of time.

When patients come to me with degenerative disc disease in their spine, our goal is to repair as much damage as possible and to restore nerve function. We then put our focus on slowing or stopping the degenerative process. Finally we teach the patient ways to reduce the stress that created the problem in the first place. For all patients, with or without degenerative disc disease, it is necessary to keep checking nerve function regularly.

Let's face it, gravity and life stresses are not on our side when it comes to health. The goal is to do everything we can to relieve the stresses so that gravity's effect on our bodies is less severe. Regular chiropractic care you. Then they have you come back when you're feeling poorly again. The good thing about relief care is that the investment in time and money is low. However, this kind of "Band-aid" help will never get you to optimum health.

Corrective care handles the basic problems behind your symptoms (the damage developed over time) and optimizes your body's structure so that your nerve system can work correctly at its best. This can get you to optimum health when combined with positive lifestyle changes. Corrective care focuses, not only on symptomatic relief by itself, but emphasizes restoring the function of the nervous system.

Supportive care provides ongoing support so that you can maintain the best life possible for as long as possible. Understand that, even while under supportive care, you may have some kind of trauma or increased stress in your life requiring further corrective care.

Corrective care combined with supportive care is an investment in your long-term health, longevity and quality of life.

If You Do Have a Bad Experience with a Chiropractor, Should You Give Up on Chiropractic Care?

If you have a situation where you don't have a good experience with one chiropractor, don't give up on chiropractic care in general. If you have a bad experience with a dentist, do you give up on dentistry? No, you find a better dentist. If you've ever had a bad experience with a mechanic, do you not take your car to a mechanic ever again? No, you find a good mechanic you like. The same is true with chiropractic care.

There are so many different styles and techniques in chiropractic that you can go to the next chiropractor and try out another approach. And if that next experience is either ineffective or uncomfortable, try another chiropractor.

How to Find and Choose a Good Chiropractor

1. **Referrals:** Ask a friend or family member for referrals and then check out the doctors recommended. Remember you are looking for a chiropractic office that will care about your betterment, evaluate you thoroughly, educate you to your understanding and effectively care for you over the long haul with retesting you along the way.

2. **Cold calls:** Use the yellow pages or your home-town service directories and call up the ones who interest you. If the receptionist answers the phone in a cheerful, happy manner, that is a good sign. The tone of the office is set by the doctor and trickles down throughout the staff. If the receptionist seems under stress, or antagonistic, you might want to move on to the next call.

3. **Websites:** Most chiropractors have websites and on their home pages present their mission statements. Check these out.

4. **Face to face interviews:** Make an appointment with a chiropractor you have heard or read about and make it clear to the receptionist that you are shopping for a chiropractor that will be just right for you. At the appointment, check out their philosophy, their evaluation procedures and how they work with the client on their plans. Find out if they treat symptoms, meaning you come in when it hurts or whether they insist on a regular care schedule to fix long term problems and subluxations. You want to work with someone who insists on creating good change—with you. You want someone who does a thorough evaluation using x-rays, tests, examination and complete medical and life incident histories. Just by feeling along the spine, the chiropractor can find different areas that are swollen, inflamed and tender or even quite painful. These areas often correlate to a lot of the problems you've been having for a long time.

5. **Seek someone who will stimulate your willingness to do something about your situation:** If a chiropractor can show you a picture of what your spine looks like after abusing it for decades, you may actually wake up and go, "Alright, I'm willing to do something about this." A good chiropractor will continually inspire you to greater health.

6. **Attend a workshop or seminar given by the chiropractor you are evaluating:** Many chiropractors give talks on lifestyle and health subjects that should inspire and motivate you. They are usually free or at a very low cost and a good way to introduce you to the office and to the chiropractor.

7. **Choose someone who is optimistic, while being realistic about how to get you better:** That is the chiropractor's job, to restore the function of your nerve system. It is not to take your money, see you a bunch of times with no or minimal results. And you want someone who is going to not just make you feel better, temporarily, but to make permanent changes.

8. **Choose someone who will retest you with x-rays, the evaluation tests and/or muscle testing:** And, who will celebrate with you and enjoy your increased health and bettered life in general.

When do you go to a chiropractor?

Traditional medical treatment, in general, is "sick" care. Chiropractic care is health care. So in answer to the question, "when to go to a chiropractor?" the answer is: when you want to get healthy and stay healthy for a lifetime.

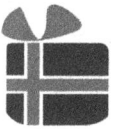

A Special Gift for You

If you live in or are visiting the Southern California area, you may call my office to arrange a chiropractic health assessment with me. For a special certificate that will save you around $200, go to www.dearoprahthebook.com, click on the special offer link, and enter dearoprah in the code box. Then just print the special certificate and bring it with you to your appointment.

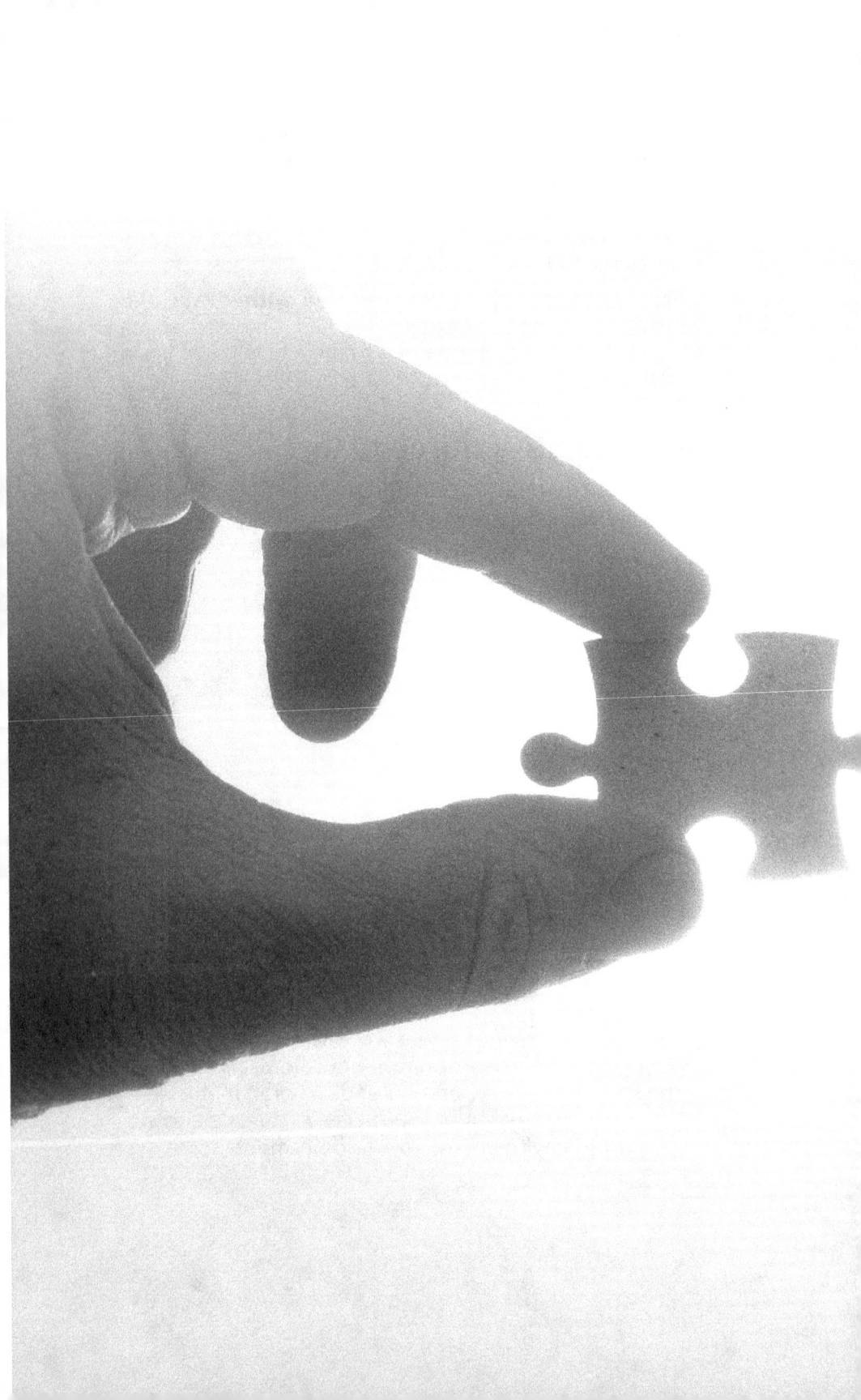

Section Three
Putting It All Together

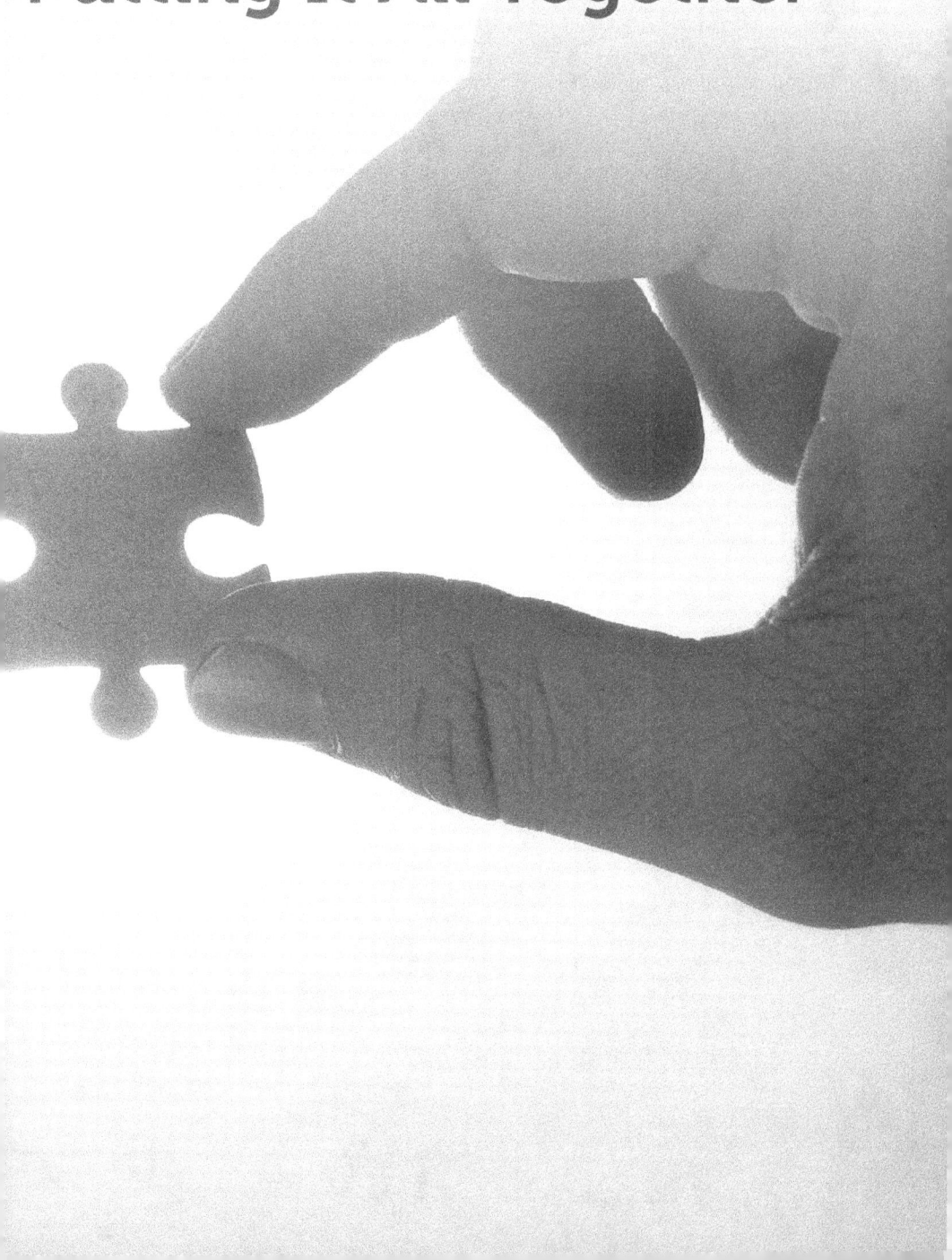

CHAPTER TWELVE
The Whole Enchilada:
Motivation, Plan, Action, Results

Y ou are motivated, you have knowledge of what to eat and not to eat, you know that the correct exercise program for you is going to play a bigger part in your life, you have decided not to put toxins on your skin, on your hair or in your body. For that matter, you are becoming more aware of toxins in the environment and resolving to do something about it. You have a greater understanding of chiropractic care and how it will benefit your life. And perhaps, best of all, you now have the tools for changing your lifestyle.

The whole point of being alive is to evolve into the complete person you were intended to be.

– Oprah

Now, let's revisit your goals. In order to have the willingness to change you have to be willing to work towards the goal and agree that it is going to be of extreme value to you to reach that goal.

If you have any hesitation about how to go about changing your lifestyle, go back to where, while reading this book, you were excited about doing this and recall what got you energized. You want to re-capture your own excitement. In other words, why did you pick up this book in the first place?

Now, if you are feeling at all overwhelmed, I want you to remember to take small steps forward mastering each milestone as you go. Start with one area, like food. Write out your ideal way of eating and what your diet will consist of. If necessary, hire a nutritionist to get you started and to monitor your progress. Weight Watchers is great for this if you have a weight challenge.

There is no substitute for your own motivation. So, we come full circle here. Revisit what you wrote in Chapter One on motivation now and may you resolve to achieve your health goals, then go about achieving them— with vigor and passion!

Only You Can Live Your Life and Live in Your Body

Let's make it simple. Only you can make your life happen, create your prosperity, be the person you know you can be. Only you can operate your body, live in it, move it around, make it be a vehicle for doing your life's work. So why not enjoy it? Why not present to the world, the most ideal you and most healthy body? It will not only benefit you, but will give immense pleasure to all who know you. You will be an inspiration to others while you live a less fettered and more fulfilled life.

Action Steps: Regarding Movement

Movement: commit to one or more of these every day

- Walk: start with three blocks, then build to five, go to ten and keep going. Find a friend who is committed to better health and do this with him or her. And/or walk your dog! If your dog is too fat, he/she is not walking/running enough!

- Join a gym and commit to going every morning for 20 minutes before work.

- Sign up with a marathon conditioning group that will help you build up stamina and strength every day. And then, run the 26 plus mile marathon and be a winner just for doing it.

- Call around and find a TurboSonic machine that you can stand on 10 to 20 minutes a day.

- Look in your yellow pages for a Boot Camp or cross fit and join it!

Action Steps: Eating

Eating: commit to doing these actions

- Eat a piece of fruit or raw vegetable before every meal.
- Eat raw foods as snacks between meals, a carrot, apple, etc.
- Go through your cupboards and donate all the processed—boxed and canned foods (that are not in your earthquake kit) or throw out old bags of flour and meal.

Action Steps: Eating

Eating: commit to doing these actions

- Find a local farmer's market and buy organic or non-sprayed produce there. At least it will be freshly picked.
- Buy a good juicer and use it.
- Commit to a fast* day once a week, where you just take off from eating and drink only water or freshly squeezed juices.
- Have a salad day, or better yet, a salad week.
- Do a three-day cleanse or longer.*
- Try going gluten free, see if you feel better.
- Buy raw milk, cheese and butter if available.
- If you cannot afford a nutritionist, read *The Maker's Diet* by Jordan Rubin, or other books recommended in my resources section.
- Take a picture of yourself in a bathing suit and post it on your refrigerator!
- Gradually, eliminate these from your diet: coffee, alcohol, refined sugars, gluten, breads, grains, sodas. Experiment, test out how you feel. Send me the results.
- If you must eat chocolate once in a while, eat only dark chocolate!
- Take a food-based multi-vitamin and start using fish oils.

* Do the fasts and diet per your nutritionist or chiropractor recommendations, as they may need to be customized for your body.

Action Steps: General Health in Daily Living

23 Ways to Increase Your Mental, Spiritual and Physical Health

1. Get a physical annually, get a good blood test and have it checked out, not only by your medical doctor, but also by an alternative doctor.

2. Research any prescription drugs you may be taking and find a medical doctor who will phase you off of them as you get better.

3. Find a chiropractor and get on a program for regular care.

4. Do your passive exercises and stretches every day & follow your exercise program.

5. Build a morning ritual. For example: review your written goals, visualize, do affirmations, and do yoga.

Action Steps: General Health in Daily Living

23 Ways to Increase Your Mental, Spiritual and Physical Health

6. Go without T.V. one or two days a week.

7. Stop listening to or reading about the news.

8. Read something inspiring every morning and/or night.

9. Have a day where you don't complain to anyone—call it your optimist day.

10. Sit quietly 20 minutes every morning.

11. De-clutter some space every day for 20 minutes.

12. Make a list of everything you've been tolerating: for example, that catch-all drawer in the kitchen, the paint on the wall that isn't right, the accumulation of emails you keep meaning to read, the cobwebs in the ceiling, the underwear with a rip! Handle something on that list each day or week.

13. Empty your mind before you go to bed. Write down things that may be bugging you, or ideas and challenges. Get them out of your head and onto the paper.

14. Watch uplifting movies with positive themes and/or read good books.

15. Write some goals that inspire you and visualize the outcome.

16. Smile. Give sincere compliments every day to show appreciation.

17. Make someone laugh, watch a comedy, go to a comedy club.

18. Talk to your pets and play with them.

19. Get a massage, or facial or manicure/pedicure, or reflexology.

20. Be adventurous: take a cooking, music or a tango class.

21. Lift somebody up who is down in the dumps.

22. Make a list of the things you've been putting off and get them done.

23. Every day, be out in nature and once a week, take a hike or extended time in nature.

WWMBMC? (What would my best me choose?)

Where you are today is based on your past choices. Where you are tomorrow is based on the choices you make today.

Unfortunately, most of us run on automatic pilot. We make choices too often based on old patterns that are detrimental to our well-being. So I've created a wrist band with the letters WWMBMC on it to help a person interrupt those patterns and remind the wearer that he/she can decide for themselves to make a healthier choice at any given moment.

We all want to catch ourselves from doing things on auto pilot that end up diminishing us, our health or progress in life. This wrist band reminds us to be our best selves and make good choices at every turn.

To get your own wristband and to get more information on how to use the wristband, go to **www.choicesformybestme.com.**

Dear Reader,

When patients come into my office, I see beyond their facades to the persons themselves, I see greatness or the possibility of greatness. It may not have come to fruition, but it is there, nonetheless. Seeing this is just plain awesome to me. My mission is to help each patient gain the health necessary to support their talents, values and dreams. I give you this book in hopes that you will care about yourself as much as I do about my patients—which is huge.

Here's the bottom line, it's your choice. Revisit your focus and goals, ask the right questions, live your values. Find a friend who will help you and hold you accountable to your new chosen lifestyle. Remember to celebrate your victories.

Here's a practical tip. Have a spouse or friend come in with you when you visit your health practitioner on the first visit. If your self-value is low then it will be helpful when your spouse says, "Just do it, I'll help you."

I give you this book in hopes that you will not only care more about yourself, but also have the tools now to manifest your self-love so that you can better give your gifts to the world. I hope that you will seek health and healing every day, every moment of your life from now on. I know that is ideal, I know we all make mistakes and slip once in a while. But today is a new day. It is filled with possibilities way beyond expectation. Love your life, live your life and live it in greater and greater health and happiness.

Love,
Dr. Dale

Dear Oprah,

You are an immense inspiration to me and to the world. I send so much admiration to you for who you are, what you do and what you will do—your legacy is beyond description. I am here to help support you both as a far-away friend and as a health practitioner. I hope this book is and will be helpful to you.

Love,
Dr. Dale

APPENDICES
APPENDIX # 1: More about Genes

In order to understand your genes, we have to understand where you've come from, because your genes have not changed much in 20,000 years! So physically, your body operates in the same way as bodies did 20,000 years ago. Our bodies have not changed, but what about our societies? The changes in our societies are the culprits in all of our major health challenges and a big reason why I wrote this book. I need to help people address these changes and get back to basics.

Your ancestors were hunter-gatherers 20,000 years ago. They had the bodies of world-class athletes. They did not have cancer, obesity, diabetes, heart disease or stroke. In order for you to express your genetic perfection, and in looking at your health, you must know what your hunter-gatherer ancestors did.

> "Genetically our bodies are virtually the same as they were at the end of the Paleolithic era some 20,000 years ago. The appearance of agriculture and domestication of animals some 10,000 years ago and the industrial revolution some 200 years ago introduced new dietary pressures for which no adaptation has been possible in such a short time span. Thus an inevitable discordance exists between our dietary intake and what our genes are suited to."
>
> **Mann, NJ. 2004** *Paleolithic Nutrition: What can we learn from the past?* **Asia Pac J Clin Nutr: 13 (Suppl): S17**

You may argue, "Yes, but they didn't live that long."

The truth is that many did die young. They died young because they were trying to kill bison and bear with sticks and stones. It was a very dangerous time for the young warrior. However, once they became elders, they lived a long, healthy life. They sent the young ones out to hunt.

Genes and Lifestyle

Today there is a whole industry studying genes to find the next new breakthrough drug to heal humankind. This is big business. They have discovered all kinds of genes that they say are responsible for the woes of our civilization. As Dr. James Chestnut says, "They even discovered a hangover gene. I know I've got it because when I drink, I get a hangover! You know what? When I don't drink, I don't get a hangover." Do you see the flaw in relying on gene therapy? It is the outside influence of the alcohol (my lifestyle choice) that triggers the gene that leads to the hangover. Wouldn't it make better sense to choose a better lifestyle and let my perfect genes be?

> "There is no doubt that some diseases, like Huntington's chorea, beta thalassemia and cystic fibrosis, can be blamed entirely on one faulty gene. But single-gene disorders affect less than two percent of the population; the vast majority of people come into this world with genes that should enable them to live a happy and healthy life. The diseases that are today's scourges—diabetes, heart disease and cancer—short circuit a happy and healthy life. These diseases, however, are not the result of a single gene, but of complex interactions among multiple genes and environmental factors."
>
> **Dr. Bruce Lipton, former medical college professor and research scientist.**

The scary part about relying on genes as a determinant of your health is seen in the example of the breast cancer gene. Many women are being convinced to lop off a breast based on their genes. It is sad and it angers me. Sure, the doctors who advise this think that they are doing what's best. However, with what you now know about genes, do you still think it is a good idea? Is it the genes or is it environmental choices? I can tell you one thing, if it was the testicular cancer gene that they were selling, no man would be lining up to get his boys cut off!

APPENDIX #2: Toxins in Cosmetics and Toiletries to Avoid

Here is a list of just a few of the "Nasties" (used with permission from **www.AbsolutelyPure.com**) lurking in your cosmetics and toiletries. Many of these are even in so-called "natural" products!

Isopropyl Alcohol: is a very drying and irritating solvent that strips your skin's moisture and natural immune barrier, making you more vulnerable to bacteria, molds and viruses. It is made from propylene, a petroleum derivative and is found in many skin and hair products, fragrances, antibacterial hand washes as well as shellac and antifreeze. It can act as a "carrier," accelerating the penetration of other harmful chemicals into your skin. In other words, it allows things to pass through the skin barrier.

Isopropyl Alcohol may promote brown spots and premature aging of skin. Inhalation or ingestion of the vapor may cause headaches, flushing, dizziness, mental depression, nausea, vomiting, narcosis, anesthesia, and even coma. An ingested dose that is fatal is one ounce or less. Other alcohols to be concerned about in skin care products are Ethyl Alcohol, Methanol, Benzyl Alcohol, SD Alcohol and denatured Alcohol.

Butyl, Ethyl, Methyl & Propyl Paraben (preservatives): are used as inhibitors of microbial growth and to extend shelf life of products. Widely used in cleansers, moisturizers, shampoos, conditioners, foundations, etc., they are known to be highly toxic. These cause gastric irritation, numbing of the mouth and many allergic reactions and skin rashes. They particularly affect asthma sufferers.

DEA, MEA & TEA (Diethanolamine, Monoethanolamine, Triethanolamine): are hormone-disrupting chemicals that can form cancer-causing nitrates and nitrosamines. These chemicals are already restricted in Europe due to known carcinogenic effects. In the United States, however, they are still used despite the fact that Americans may be exposed to them on a daily basis with products such as shampoos, shaving creams and bubble baths.

Diazolidinyl Urea & Imidazolidinyl Urea: are just two of many preservatives that often release formaldehyde. Yes, formaldehyde, the substance they used in your biology class to preserve dead frogs! Formaldehyde may cause joint pain, skin reactions, allergies, depression, headaches, chest pains, ear infections, chronic fatigue, dizziness, and loss of sleep. Diazolidinyl Urea & Imidazolidinyl Urea are used in cleansers, toners, moisturizers etc. Exposure may also irritate the respiratory system, trigger heart palpitations or asthma, and aggravate coughs and colds. Other possible side effects include weakening the immune system and cancer. These are the most commonly used preservatives after the parabens.

FD&C Color Pigments: are synthetic colors made from coal tar used in cosmetics like eye shadow, blusher, foundation and lipstick, containing heavy metal salts that deposit toxins onto the skin, causing sensitivity and irritation. Absorption of certain colors can cause depletion of oxygen in the body and even cause death. Animal studies have shown almost all of them to be carcinogenic.

Synthetic Fragrances: when tested, can indicate the presence of up to four thousand separate ingredients, many toxic or carcinogenic. Symptoms reported to the FDA include headaches, dizziness, allergic rashes, skin discoloration, violent coughing and vomiting, and skin irritation. Clinical observation proves fragrances can affect the central nerve system, causing depression, hyperactivity, irritability, inability to cope, and other behavioral changes.

Mineral Oil, Liquid Paraffin (Paraffinum Liquidum): are all petroleum by-products that coat the skin like plastic wrap, clogging the pores. These interfere with your skin's ability to eliminate toxins, thus promoting acne and other disorders. These may cause skin discoloration and they slow down skin function and cell development, resulting in premature aging. They are used in many products because they are cheap. Baby oil is 100% mineral oil!

Petrolatum & Petroleum Jelly: mineral oil jelly, like mineral oil, interferes with the body's own natural moisturizing mechanism, leading to dry skin and chapping. These appear in lip gloss, lipstick and lip balm. We are being sold products that actually create the very conditions they claim to alleviate. Manufacturers use it because it is unbelievably cheap.

Polyethylene Glycol (PEG): is a potentially carcinogenic petroleum ingredient that can alter and reduce the skin's natural moisture factor. This could increase the appearance of aging and leave you more vulnerable to bacteria. It is also used in cleansers to dissolve oil and grease. It adjusts the melting point and thickens products. It is also used in caustic spray-on oven cleaners.

Propylene Glycol (PG) & Butylene Glycol: are gaseous hydrocarbons, which in a liquid state act as "surfactants" (wetting agents and solvents). They easily penetrate the skin and can weaken protein and cellular structure. Commonly used in cleansers, moisturizers, body lotions, foundations, etc., they are also used in industrial anti-freeze and hydraulic brake fluid! PG is strong enough to remove barnacles from boats!

The EPA (Environmental Protection Agency) considers PG so toxic that it requires workers to wear protective gloves, clothing and goggles and to dispose of any PG solutions by burying them in the ground. Because PG penetrates the skin so quickly, the EPA warns against skin contact to prevent consequences such as brain, liver, and kidney abnormalities. But there isn't even a warning label on products such as stick deodorants, where the concentration is greater than in most industrial applications! They are also used in some salad dressings. Yuk!

Sodium Lauryl Sulfate (SLS) & Sodium Laureth Sulfate (SLES): are industrial detergents and surfactants that pose serious health threats. They are used in car washes, garage floor cleaners and engine degreasers and in

90% of personal care products that foam, such as toothpaste, bubble bath, shampoo, bath and shower gel, facial cleansers and hand-washes because they are cheap. A small amount generates a large amount of foam, and when salt is added, it thickens to give the illusion of being rich and concentrated.

Animals exposed to SLS experience eye damage, depression, labored breathing, diarrhea, severe skin irritation, and even death. Young eyes may not develop properly if exposed to SLS because proteins are dissolved. SLS may also damage the skin's immune system by causing layers to separate and inflame. When combined with other chemicals, SLS can be transformed into nitrosamines, a potent class of carcinogens. Your body may retain SLS for up to five days, during which time it may enter and maintain residual levels in the heart, liver, lungs, and brain.

Triclosan: is a synthetic "antibacterial" ingredient with a chemical structure similar to Agent Orange! The EPA (Environmental Protection Agency) registers it as a pesticide, giving it high scores as a risk to both human health and the environment. It is classified as a chloroprene, a class of chemicals suspected of causing cancer in humans. Its manufacturing process may produce dioxin, a powerful hormone-disrupting chemical with toxic effects measured in parts per trillion; that is only one drop in 300 Olympic-size swimming pools!

Hormone Disruptors: pose enormous long-term chronic health risks by interfering with the way hormones perform, such as changing genetic material, decreasing fertility and sexual function, and fostering birth defects. It can temporarily de-activate sensory nerve endings, so contact with it often causes little or no pain. Internally, it can lead to cold sweats, circulatory collapse, and convulsions. Stored in body fat, it can accumulate to toxic levels, damaging the liver, kidneys and lungs, and can cause paralysis, suppression of immune function, brain hemorrhages, and heart problems.

Tufts University School of Medicine (Boston) says that triclosan is capable of forcing the emergence of "super bugs" that it cannot kill. Its widespread use in popular antibacterial cleansers, toothpastes, mouthwashes and household products may have nightmare implications for our future.

Phthalates: (pronounced tha - lates) can be absorbed through the skin, inhaled as fumes, ingested when they contaminate food or when children bite or suck on toys, and are inadvertently but directly administered to patients from some PVC (polyvinyl chloride or vinyl) medical devices. Hundreds of animal studies have shown that phthalates can damage the liver, kidneys, lungs and the reproductive system, especially the developing testes. Phthalates are found in many leading beauty care products, including hair spray, deodorant, nail polish and perfume that you may be using everyday.

APPENDIX #3: Vibrational Therapy

The Russian space program came up with the technology called **vibrational therapy**. There is a particular model called the TurboSonic. And if you look at any vibrational device, the main thing to understand is that you want a straight up-and-down motion as opposed to any side-to-side motion. Because when it becomes a side-to-side motion, it tends to tear up your knees and tear up your hips and tear up your ankles. However, with a straight up-and-down, it simulates gravity and that allows you to contract and relax.

The TurboSonic uses sound waves to move a plate up-and-down. This plate knocks you off balance so you have to contract muscles in order to stay balanced. And this happens really fast, so it's contract and relax, contract and relax. It happens so fast that, actually, if you're on it for ten minutes, it's like you did over an hour of cardio-vascular exercise. So it's a very quick way to get your aerobics in. And, as the frequency changes on this machine, it will actually work out different areas of your body. One frequency will do legs, one frequency will do stomach. And the other cool thing that it does is it actually exercises your face, so it can reduce your wrinkles. It's one of the few exercise technologies that works your face muscles so they contract and relax. It increases bone density and decreases the effects of stress. It increases human growth hormone, dopamine and serotonin secretion, lowers cortisol and epinephrine secretion and enhances circulation, all of which counteract the effects of stress on the body and spirit.

Benefits of TurboSonic Vibrational Exercise

- Gives you over an hour of cardiovascular workout in about ten minutes on the machine
- Can decrease the effects of stress
- Increases bone density
- Increases human growth hormone, dopamine and serotonin secretion
- Lowers cortisol and epinephrine secretion
- Enhances circulation
- Can reduce facial wrinkles
- As the frequency changes on this machine, it will actually work out different areas of your body.

Contra-indications for TurboSonic Vibrational Exercise

If any of the conditions listed below apply to you, consult your physician or competent healthcare practitioner who is familiar with whole body vibration therapy before using the TurboSonic Vibration Therapy Trainer.

Consult your healthcare practitioner if you have:

- A serious cardiovascular condition
- A pacemaker or other electrical implant
- Had a recent surgery
- Acute thrombosis
- Had hip, knee or other joint replacements
- Epilepsy
- Severe diabetes
- Acute hernia or discopathy
- Severe migraines
- A tumor
- A recently placed IUD, or metal pins or plates
- Or, if you are pregnant

Movement stimulates human growth hormone and several other things to help you stay young and rejuvenated. This is a fabulous way, if you stand on the TurboSonic once or twice a day, to get tons of aerobic exercise and be healthy in a short amount of time. As stated above, it is important to check with your health care professional because there are some contra-indications to this kind of force being put on your body. But I highly recommend the TurboSonic because I like the idea of sound waves as opposed to mechanical vibrational therapy machines that tend to break more easily.

APPENDIX #4: More information on how to find where you are on the Health Continuum

Find a Creating Wellness Center (www.creatingwellness.com) and make an appointment for an assessment. It's really amazing and insightful. This is why I decided to purchase the equipment and the NASA Certified program for our office.

This is from the Creating Wellness Website:

Your journey begins with your Creating Wellness Assessment. Using state-of-the-art, scientific technology and a comprehensive lifestyle questionnaire, our assessment evaluates your wellness in each of the three dimensions (Physical, Bio-Chemical, and Psychological). The Creating Wellness Assessment measures and records such factors as nervous system function, body composition, stress response--and over 50 other factors that are crucial indicators of your over-all wellness. This evaluation allows us to focus on the specific needs that must be met in order for you to increase your wellness in all three dimensions.

Our powerful computer software uses your assessment to calculate your Wellness Quotient. Your Wellness Quotient is a snapshot of your overall state of wellness — think of it as your Wellness IQ. It is the sum total of your present Physical, Bio-Chemical and Psychological well-being and the foundation from which you will begin to create wellness in your life.

APPENDIX # 5: Chiropractic Care and Children

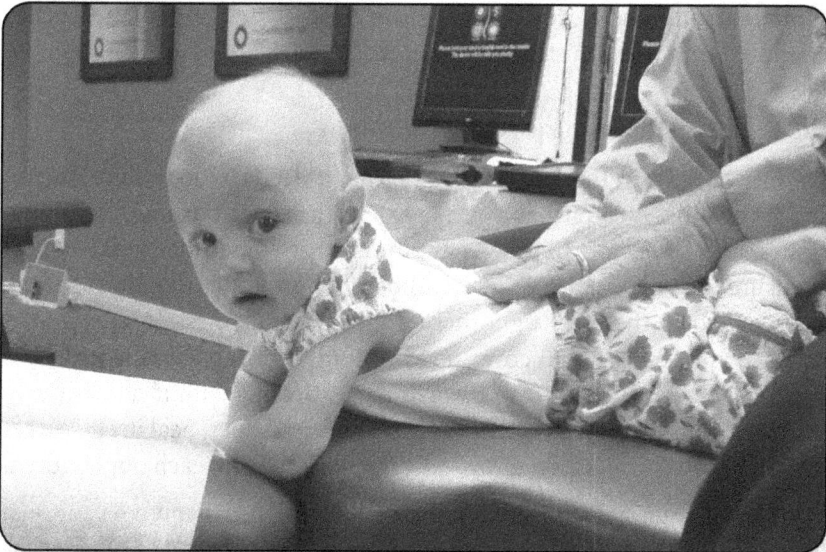

Why I'm So Glad My Daughter Is a Chiropractic Kid
By Barbara Rousey
I know that chiropractic is about more than pain relief.

Those of us who have had the good fortune to get chiropractic care on a regular basis realize that it keeps us healthier, happier, and better able to handle the stresses of life. Sure, we still experience injuries and soreness on occasion. This is normal. But we know that chiropractic keeps our systems working efficiently so that we heal correctly.

Many people, even those who recognize the benefits of chiropractic wellness care for themselves, don't think it has anything to offer children.

They go back to the idea of pain relief, particularly back pain, and assume that their child has no pain to alleviate.

I know that even at four months, Evan has had subluxations. The birth process, being held and passed from person to person, riding in the car and stroller, and exercising new wobbly muscles, all can cause subluxations. Soon she'll be sitting up (and falling), crawling (and bumping into things), walking (and falling some more). Chiropractic care will keep her free from the problems that can develop when these subluxations go uncared for into adulthood. Her nervous system, and therefore her entire body, will grow without interference.

We also know that chiropractic care keeps the immune system functioning better. Evan will have fewer colds, ear infections, and other common childhood ailments. When she does get sick, she will heal faster than her peers without chiropractic care.

She will learn the "natural first" philosophy.

Evan will learn that the body does what it needs to do to fight disease and get healthy. A cough has a purpose. Diarrhea has a purpose. Vomiting, rashes, and fever, too. These "symptoms" that sometimes make us feel awful are the body's way of fighting those foreign things that don't belong in us. We help the body fight these things naturally first. Medicine has its place, but if it's only to cover up symptoms that can actually delay the healing process, and so, it's not worth it. By dealing with it naturally, we learn and reinforce the idea that the body can, and does, heal itself. We get stronger in the process. And this is a valuable lesson to teach our children.

We, and our children, are bombarded by the media and conventional thinking that there's a pill for every symptom. I'm sure you've noticed the advertisements of happy people on some sort of drug, and it's not even clear what the drug is actually for. But the people sure do look happy! For many children, there has been a constant stream of drugs, beginning with antibiotics, cough medicine, cold medicine, behavior medicine. And it is no wonder that teens begin experimenting with illegal drugs. There is no clear line between illicit and prescription drugs. The message is the same: Take this drug and you'll feel better. Our daughter will grow up knowing that her body is a magnificent, self-healing, self-regulating instrument to be treated with care.

She'll avoid the common problems that adults face.

Just ask Dr. Ellwein. Many, many issues that bring people into a chiropractic office are not new injuries. Some of them have been going on since childhood. That time you fell off of your bike? Tripped over something? Ran into something? Rough-housed with a friend? Fought with a sibling? Played sports? Carried a heavy backpack? When we're kids, our healing mechanisms work pretty fast. The body compensates for injuries quickly, and we easily forget them. Then we come in for care as adults with health issues, and they take a long time to handle. Chiropractic kids like Evan will heal more quickly and, as adults, will be spared from many of the challenges their parents faced.

She will also learn the value of taking care of herself. So often, as adults, we get caught up in the day-to-day details and lose sight of the big picture. We forget to take care of ourselves until a health crisis gets our attention by interfering with our lives. Chiropractic is an important part of making one's health a priority, deserving regular attention, even when we "feel fine." I want my daughter to thrive, to enjoy and appreciate life, not just survive and get by.

Chiropractic is Safe

A chiropractic adjustment for a child looks much different than one for an adult. Adjustments are performed using about the same amount of pressure that you would use to check the ripeness of a tomato. Because they don't have all of the muscle tension accompanying subluxations that adults do, the adjustment is extremely gentle and very effective. Chiropractic is a natural, non-invasive health care system whose safety record cannot be beat. I am so glad that chiropractic is Evan's primary form of health care, from before birth, and that she is on her way to a strong, happy, healthy life.

For more information on Children and Chiropractic, go to The International Chiropractic Pediatric Association's website:

www.icpa4kids.org

Resources

Great Websites

mercola.com – The number one health reference on the internet

icpa4kids.org – Chiropractic for kids resource

creatingwellness.com – To find a Creating Wellness Center

vita-test.com - a great symptom based nutritional test

Other Great Books on Wellness

The Wellness and Prevention Paradigm – Dr. James L. Chestnut, B.Ed., MSc., D.C., CCWP

Discover Wellness: How Staying Healthy Can Make You Rich – Drs. Bob Hoffman and Jason Deitch

The 100 Year Lifestyle – Dr. Eric Plasker

The Power of Self-Healing: Unlock Your Natural Healing Potential in 21 Days! – Dr. Fabrizio Mancini

Chiropractic First – Dr. Terry A. Rondberg

Eat Well Books

The Paleo Diet: Lose Weight and Get Healthy by Eating the Foods You Were Designed to Eat – Dr. Loren Cordain

The Maker's Diet – Jordan S. Rubin

High Quality Supplement Companies

innatechoice.com
standardprocess.com
metagenics.com
purposenutrition.com

bioticsresearch.com

Emotional Health Books

Biology of Belief: Unleashing the Power of Consciousness, Matter, and Miracles – Dr. Bruce Lipton

The Breakthrough Experience: A Revolutionary New Approach to Personal Transformation – Dr. John F. Demartini

The Six Pillars of Self-Esteem: The Definitive Work on Self-Esteem by the Leading Pioneer in the Field – Dr. Nathaniel Branden

Any of the *Chicken Soup for the Soul* books – Jack Canfield and Mark Victor Hansen

About the Author

Dr. Dale Ellwein is a wellness lifestyle specialist. He received his doctorate in Chiropractic from Life Chiropractic College West in Hayward, California in 1991, and did advance studies with Dr. James L. Chestnut earning his Chiropractic Wellness Professional Certification.

Dr. Ellwein inspires people of all ages to achieve peak performance, focus, mental acuity, and amazing health. He teaches simple, proven systems that inspire his patients to eat, move and think in ways that support their longevity and vital, healing nature.

Using the essential combination of lifestyle management and advanced chiropractic care, Dr. Ellwein has helped thousands of individuals overcome aches, pains, and diseases, and improve their overall quality of life. His proven program has been shown to restore health and healing in the bodies of his patients—often leading to long, inspired, joy-filled lives.

Dr. Ellwein practices in Southern California, where he lives with his wife, Barbara, two children, three dogs and six chickens. He conducts lecture series in his office, Standing Tall Chiropractic, and several of his talks, videos, and articles can be found on the internet.

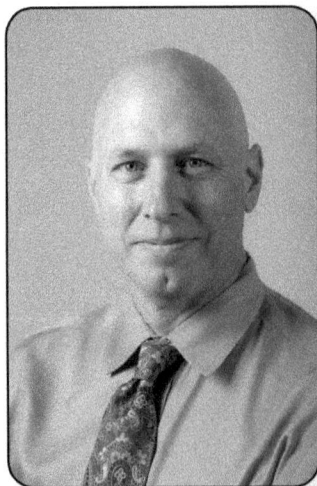

www.ingramcontent.com/pod-product-compliance
Lightning Source LLC
Chambersburg PA
CBHW060904280326
41934CB00007B/1184